Y.-C. Zhang K. Kawai (Eds.)

Precancerous Conditions and Lesions of the Stomach

With 46 Figures and 19 Tables

Springer-Verlag
Berlin Heidelberg New York
London Paris Tokyo
Hong Kong Barcelona
Budapest

Professor Dr. Ying-Chang Zhang
Deputy Director
Cancer Institute of China Medical University
5-3 Najing Street, Heping District
Shenyang, 110001, People's Republic of China

Professor Dr. Keiichi Kawai
Department of Preventive Medicine
Kyoto Prefectural University of Medicine
Kawaramachi Hirokoji
Kamigyo-ku, Kyoto, 602, Japan

ISBN 3-540-55443-2 Springer-Verlag Berlin Heidelberg New York
ISBN 0-387-55443-2 Springer-Verlag New York Berlin Heidelberg

Library of Congress Cataloging-in-Publication Data. Precancerous conditions and lesions of the stomach/ Y.-C. Zhang, K. Jawai (eds.). p. cm. Includes bibliographical references and index. ISBN 3-540-55443-2 (alk. paper).—ISBN 0-387-55443-2 (alk. paper) 1. Stomach—Precancerous conditions. I. Zhang, Y.-C. (Ying-Chang), 1923– II. Kawai, Keiichi, 1932– . [DNLM: 1. Precancerous Conditions. 2. Stomach Neoplasms—diagnosis. WI 320 P9225] RC280.S8P73 1992 616.99′433071—dc20 DNLM/DLC for Library of Congress 92-2329 CIP

Printed in Hong Kong

Typesetting: Best-set Typesetter Ltd., Hong Kong
25/3130-5 4 3 2 1 0—Printed on acid-free paper

Preface

The strategy adopted for the control of gastric cancer, involving both primary and secondary prevention, is very important. The development of epidemio-etiological studies and the adoption of many measures for reducing or blocking risk factors as well as increasing protective factors have reduced the incidence of gastric cancer in many countries. For example, in such countries as the USA and Finland, the incidence of gastric cancer has decreased strikingly during the last few decades. Even in Japan, whose people are among those at highest risk from this disease, the incidence of gastric cancer has decreased. In China, too (northeast China, a high risk area), the incidence of gastric cancer has tended to decrease in comparison with the situation that prevailed 15 years ago, according to recent reports.

Although the incidence of gastric cancer has decreased, or is decreasing, in many areas of the world, the background of the diseases to which gastric mucosa is subject, i.e., the different gastric diseases and precursors of gastric cancer, in inhabitants of the high risk areas in particular is not yet clearly known. Studies of precursors of gastric cancer are not merely of academic or theoretical importance, but are valuable in that they contribute to the development of primary prevention in practice.

In clinical practice, secondary prevention, i.e., early detection and early treatment, particulary the former, plays an important role at present. It is known, for example, that a 5-year survival rate after surgical treatment for early gastric cancer may be the result of early detection and early treatment made possible by advances in examination techniques. Studies on precursors of gastric cancer have also produced many useful contributions from pathologists and gastroenterologists. Many studies in this field have been published but the subject has not been fully clarified. I believe that the studies presented here may help in many ways to promote the early detection of gastric cancer.

In addition, conservative (including chemical) and surgical treatment for many precancerous conditions or precancerous lesions of the stomach are being carried out, and gratifying results have been achieved. In a sense, this has also played a primary prevention tole in gastric cancer. Follow-up studies of many precancerous lesions or gastric dysplasias have up to now been looked upon as important ways both of promoting early detection of gastric cancer and clarifying the natural history of precancerous changes. In the author's experience, however, repeated endoscopic examinations and biopsies during follow-up for very small precancerous changes in the gastric mucosa have not been particularly successful as aids to the rediscovery and diagnosis of previously recognized lesions, except in the case of particular precancerous lesions, e.g., the protruding type or adenomatous type of gastric dysplasia. Therefore, it is necessary that more precise techniques or methods be developed for the study of these kinds of pathological changes of the gastric mucosa. It is expected that markers for detecting these pathological changes microscopically or even for endoscopic screening will be developed. More attention should be paid, too, to animal experiments involving the induction of precancerous changes in the stomach, as it has been reported by some authors that many previously unaccepted "causes" of precancerous change in the gastric mucosa are now accepted.

Another point which we believe to be significant is that different etiologic factors prevail in some of the different high risk areas of the world, while the mucosal changes, including the precancerous lesions and spectrum of gastric diseases of the inhabitants, probably differ also from area to area. Two high risk areas, Hokkaido in northern Japan and Liaodong Panisula in northeast China, serve as examples of this. A common findings in the gastric mucosae of the inhabitants of the former town is chronic gastritis with striking intestinal metaplasia, whereas in the latter town chronic gastritis with erosions and regenerations is prominent. This phenomenon affirms the need for geographic or epidemiologic pathological study of the precancerous changes of the stomach in order that the characteristics and natural history of these lesions of the stomach might be clarified.

Yin-Chang Zhang
Keiichi Kawai

Contents

List of Contributors

Addresses are given at the beginning of the respective contribution.

1 General Remarks

Y.-C. Zhang

Although the incidence and mortality of stomach cancer are decreasing world-wide, it is still the main cancer in many countries [7, 8]. In Japan, the mortality rate from this cancer is 41.39/100 000, and about 25% of all malignant neoplasms are stomach cancers [7, 8, 21, 26]. In China, too, stomach cancer ranks first among all cancers, the mortality rate being 23.86/100 000, and about 160 000 people die of this cancer in China each year [18].

In the strategy for cancer control, primary prevention is of fundamental importance. In fact, many effective results have already been achieved owing to, for example, environmental improvements, and a greater general understanding among People of the need to refrain from those things which put them at risk and to take steps which provide protection against stomach cancer. At present, however, secondary prevention measure, i.e., early detection and early treatment, also provide practical help in bringing about a decrease in the number of deaths caused by stomach cancer. In other words, more patients may be cured if more stomach cancers are detected at an early stage. The early detection of these cancers owes much, in many countries, to the increasing efficiency of examination techiques for gastric diseases; thus, the ratio of stomach cancers found early to those identified later is steadily increasing. At the same time, the 5-year survival rate of patients treated surgically for stomach cancer is also increasing. To improve the outlook still further, the study of precursors of stomach cancer may provide a valuable basis for preventing the development of stomach cancers or detecting these cancers in their early stages.

Although studies of the precursors of stomach cancer still continue, some confusion still attends the concept, criteria, and natural history of these gastric conditions. Fortunately, many important achievements have been made by groups carrying out these studies, and, since 1978, important concepts have been proposed by many study groups [11, 13, 14, 16]. As a result of their work, precursors of stomach cancer have been classified as (a) precancerous conditions or (b) precancerous lesions. Precancerous conditions are clinical entities, i.e., chronic atrophic gastritis, gastric ulcer,

Cancer Institute of China Medical University, 5-3 Nanjing Street, Heping District, Shenyang 110001, P. R. China

Ying-Chan Zhang/Keiichi Kawai (Eds.)
Precancerous Conditions and Lesions of the Stomach

gastric polyp, Ménétrier's disease, gastric stump, etc., from which stomach cancers are likely to develop. The precancerous lesion, by contrast, is a pathological change, i.e., a change out of which stomach cancer may well develop. In other words, malignant transformation can occur in these lesions.

It is known that stomach cancer develops more frequently in precanceous conditions than in other gastric diseases because precancerous lesions usually exist with the former. Clinicians, therefore, regard the clinical assessment of the malignant potential of a precancerous condition in a patient as both desirable and practical. But one clinician's or pathologist's understanding of precancerous conditions and precancerous lesions sometimes differs from that of others. The precancerous condition, as a clinical concept, should be treated carefully as sometimes a precancerous lesion exists with in it. Chronic gastric ulcer was once looked upon as a common precancerous condition, whereas in recent years, controversy has surrounded its malignant potential; there are two very different views about whether or not, from this common condition, gastric cancer may develop. Chronic gastric ulcer was traditionally cited in many textbooks as being a precursor of gastric cancer. In recent years, however, many clinicians and pathologists have observed, on the basis of their own endoscopic and histopathological studies, that there is little or no inevitable relationship between chronic gastric ulcer and gastric cancer [16, 17, 19, 20]. It is necessary, therefore, to clarify this.

Most pathologists and clinicians know that chronic atrophic gastritis is one of the antecedants of gastric cancer [1, 16, 23]. Follow-up studies have revealed that in about 10% of patients suffering from chronic atrophic gastritis cancer has occurred during the following 10–20 years. What kind of histopathological changes, or, more concretely, what kind of epithelial changes, may lead to malignant transformation in chronic atrophic gastritis? From the pathologist's standpoint, detailed studies of this condition are his or her professional responsibility.

Intestinal metaplasia of gastric mucosa, usually accompanied by chronic atrophic gastritis, was traditionally looked upon as a precancerous lesion or precancerous condition [6, 25]. Since 1978, however, many types of intestinal metaplasia have been classified according to the characteristics of mucins secreted by the metaplastic epithelia; much enthusiasm was shown in this study field for a period of time. Now a majority of pathologists agree that the incomplete colonic type of intestinal metaplasia has a close relationship with gastric cancer, or they look upon it as a precancerous lesion [6, 22, 25]. Coincidentally, some types of intestinal metaplasia, e.g., type IIB of Jass (see Chap. 5, "Classification of IM"), usually showed frankly epithelial dysplasia and were classified as one type of gastric dysplasia.

Since the adenomatous and cryptal types of gastric dysplasia proposed by Zhang both consist of the intestinal type of epithelia, it is appropriate to correlate some types of intestinal metaplasia with gastric dysplasia.

As for the gastric polyp, its adenomatous type was reported by many authors to be subject to a greater degree of malignant change because of its lining of dysplastic epithelia, but recent reports have noted that malignant transformations were also found in hyperplastic polyps. It is not strange that dysplastic epithelia might exist in the latter [11, 12].

As explained in the literature, sumilarities between the adenomatous polyp (or adenoma) and the dysplasia of adenomatous type (or atypical epithelial lesion) sometimes confused readers because both of these pathologic conditions usually had protruded and well defined foci. Some of the latter, however, are in the form of flat elevated patches whereas the former are usually hemispherical and of a pedunculated polypoid shape macroscopically. While their naked shapes are somewhat different, their histopathologic attributes are alike. Adenomatous polyp and dysplasia of adenomatous type have similarities, then, but are not synonymous, e.g., some of the latter showed depressed shape macroscopically and microscopically.

Gastric dysplasia, or epithelial dysplasia of the stomach, is regarded as a precancerous lesion by most pathologists today. The pathologic changes associated with these dysplasias may be found in many conditions of the gastric mucosa and many types have been proposed [2, 5, 11, 13, 14, 16, 24, 31, 33].

Evaluation of the grade of atypism or the malignant potential of a dysplastic lesion is another problem for pathologists. Three grades have been used in practice: mild, moderate, and severe, or grades I, II, and III. In fact, these categories are somewhat artificial because a dysplastic change and its atypism are transitional. Therefore, grading for a given case of gastric dysplasia has usually varied from one pathologist to another and owed something to a particular pathologist's personal experience or understanding of these lesions, this despite the fact that many morphological descriptions for grading dysplastic changes have been cited in papers, booklets and textbooks. In a workshop on gastric dysplasia and related lesions held in San Miniato, Italy, by the International Study Group on Gastric Cancer (ISGGC) in 1982, many slides of gastric dysplasia contributed by participants were evaluated for grades of atypism by skilled pathologists in this study field [12]. Identical slides received different evaluations and gradings from different pathologists. In some cases one slide received separate evaluations ranging from nondysplasia, to severe dysplasia or even malignant lesion. This situation underlines the need for more objective criteria in the grading of gastric dysplasia.

In recent years, there have been two primary aspects in the search for objectivity in the grading of gastric dysplasias: (a) the attempt by many pathologists to find some markers specific to stomach cancer which will be useful for evaluating the atypism of gastric dysplasia, and (b) quantitative measurement of pathologic changes by morphometric techniques.

Immunohistochemical staining for some markers has been reported in evaluation of the atypism of gastric epithelia [3, 4, 28]. Some are such well known antigens as carcino-embryonic antigens (CEA), ABH isoantigens, Lewis antigens, lectins, enzymes, and many laboratories' own antibodies (monoclonal or polyclonal) or biologic reagents. It was found, genereally, that the degree to which some of these markers expressed was consistent with the severity of atypism. Although the markers were not specific, in normal gastric epithelia they usually demonstrated polarity in the epithelial cells, while in malignant epithelia loss of polarity in the distribution of the markers was a common finding. Not all the markers reported were, however, sufficiently specific to be used as clinicopathological indexes for practically evaluating the grade of epithelial dysplasia.

With the advent of more advanced morphometric techniques, objective indexes for evaluating dysplastic grades have been proposed [27, 29, 30]. DNA content in normal epithelium, and cancer cell and its intermediate dysplastic epithelium, were measured by microspectrometry and flow cytometry. In the range of normal to dysplastic and malignant epithelia, except for the diploidy of normal epithelium, tetraploidy and aneuploidy are looked upon as signs of atypism or malignancy of the epitherlium, but there is usually overlapping of the various grades of dysplastic change, as is also the case with cancers. Some authors believe that if aneuploidy appears in a dysplastic lesion the malignant nature of the lesion is established.

Autoimage analysis systems have been used to evaluate grades of atypism of gastric dysplasia in recent years. Many quantitative measurement indexes for architectural and cellular atypism have been designed and are used in clinicopathological examination. These morphometric studies may at least help to standardize to a great extent, the objective criteria of gastric dysplasia.

Among the precursors of gastric cancer, environmental and host factors should be fully taken into account. Geographic/pathologic studies have revealed a relationship between some histopathologic types of stomach cancer and the patients' environments. For instance, more cases of intestinal-type stomach cancer have been occurring in high-risk areas despite its decrease at a faster rate than diffuse types of stomach cancer in other areas, due to improvements in variour environmental factors including diet. Since the diffuse types of stomach cancer have been maintaining their former incidence, the incidence of these cancers probably has little or nothing to do with environmental change [9, 15]. The author's recent comparative, etiologic and histopathologic studies of Chinese and Japanese people living in high risk areas of their respective countries [10, 32, 34], has revealed that one country's spectrum of gastric mucosal changes is different from the other's. Chronic gastritis with intestinal metaplasia was found more commonly in Japanese inhabitants, while in Chinese inhabitants active chronic gastritis accompanying epithelial degenerations and erosions was more striking. Gastric dysplasia of regenerative type was also striking in Chinese inhabitants. Therefore, I propose that in the study of the precursors of stomach cancer epidemiologic or geographic/pathologic factors should be considered fully.

References

1. Correa P (1983) Chronic atrophic gastritis as a precursor of cancer. In: Sherlock P, et al. (eds) Precancerous lesions of the gastrointestinal tract. Raven, New York, pp 145–153
2. Cuello C, Correa P, Zarama G, Lopez J, Murrar J, Gordillo G (1979) Histopathology of gastric dysplasia. Am J Pathol 3:491–500
3. Filipe MI, Barbatis C, Sandey A, Ma J (1988) Expression of intestinal mucin antigens in the gastric epithelium and its relationship with malignancy. Hum Pathol 19:19–26
4. Hakkinen IPT, Heinonen R, Inbeg MV, Jarvi OH, Vaajalahti P, Viikari S (1980) Clinicopathological study of gastric cancers and precancerous states detected by fetal sulfoglycoprotein antigen screening. Cancer Res 40:4308–4312
5. Hirota T, Itabashi M, Takizawa C, Kim BK (1987) Clinico-pathological characteristics of gastric adenoma and its significance as a precancerous lesion. Stomach Intest 22:657–664
6. Jass JR (1980) Role of intestinal metaplasia in the histogenesis of gastric carcinoma. J Clin Pathol 33:801–810
7. Kurihara M, Aoki K, Hisamichi S (1980) Cancer mortality statistics in the world (UICC, 1950–1979). University of Nagoya Press, Nagoya
8. Kurihara M, Aoki K, Hisamichi S (1989) Cancer mortality statistics in the world (UICC, 1950–1985). University of Nagoya Press, Nagoya
9. Lauren P (1965) The two histological main types of gastric carcinoma, diffuse and so-called intestinal type carcinoma. An attempt at a histo-clinical classification. Acta Pathol Microbiol Scand 64:31–49
10. Lin HZ, Zhang YC (1987) Geographic pathology of stomach cancer in China-review. In: Wada T, Aoki K, Yachi A (eds) Current status of cancer research in Asia, The Middle East and other countries. University of Nagoya Press, Nagoya, pp 41–49
11. Ming SC (1984) Precursors of gastric cancer. Praeger, New York
12. Ming SC, Goldman H (1965) Gastric polyps: a histogenetic classification and its relation to carcinoma. Cancer 18:721–726
13. Ming SC, Bajitai A, Correa Elster K, Jarvi OH, Nagayo T, Stemmermann GN (1984) Gastric dysplasia: significance and pathologic criteria. Cancer 54:1794–1801
14. Morson BC, Sobin LH, Grundmann E, Johansen A, Nagayo T, Serck-Hanssen A (1980) Precancerous conditions and epithelial dysplasia in the stomach. J Clin Pathol 33:711–721
15. Munoz N, Connelly P (1971) Time trends of intestinal and diffuse type of stomach cancer in the United States. Int J Cancer 8:158–164
16. Nagayo T (1986) Histogenesis and precursors of human gastric cancer. Springer, Berlin Heidelberg New York
17. Nakamura K (1982) Structure of the gastric cancer (in Japanese). Igaku-Shion, Tokyo
18. Office of Prevention and Treatment for Neoplasms of the Ministry of Health (1979) Survey of mortalities of malignant neoplasms in China. People's Health Publish House, Beijing
19. Oota K (1963) Role of gastric ulcer in the causation of gastric cancer in Japan: a histopathological study of 3000 gastrectomy materials. Acta Unio Int Contou Cancrum 19:1208–1209
20. Oota K (1976) Early phase of development of human gastric cancer. Gann Monogr Cancer Res 18:77–83
21. Segi M, Tominaga S, Aoki K, Fujimoto I (1981) Cancer mortality and morbidity statistics. Gann Monogr Cancer Res 26
22. Segura DI, Montero C (1983) Histochemical characterization of different types of intestinal metaplasia in gastric mucosa. Cancer 52:498–503
23. Siurala M, Varis K, Wiljasalo M (1960) Studies of patients with atrophic gastritis: a 10–15 year follow-up. Scand J Gastroenterol 1:40–48
24. Sugano H (1972) The pathological morphology of the borderline lesion in digestive tract: atypical epithelium of the stomach (in Japanese). Gan No Rinsho 18:834–842

25. Teglbjarg PS, Nielson HO (1978) "Small intestinal type" and "colonic type" intestinal metaplasia of the human stomach. Acta Pathol Microbiol Scand 86:351–355
26. Tominaga S, Kurishi T, Aoki K, Fijimoto I (1982) Cancer mortality and morbidity statistics in Japan. In: Aoki K, Tominaga S, Hirayama T, Hirota Y (eds) Cancer prevention in developing countries. University of Nagoya Press, Nagoya
27. Wang RN, Zhao ML, Su BH, Xiao SD, Jiang SJ (1988) A model assessment of gastric precancerous lesions by morphometric analysis. Chin Med J 101:403–409
28. Yachi A (1988) Cancer of the digestive organs and cancer markers (in Japanese). Health Publish House, Tokyo
29. Yen RF, Zhang YC, Wu YQ (1987) Morphological measurement for diagnosis of gastric dysplasia (Engl Abstr). Zhonghua Zhongliu Zazhi (Chin J Oncol) 9:401–404
30. Yen RF, Zhang YC, Wu YQ (1989) Morphometric indexes and computerized diagnosis of gastric dysplasia. Proc Chin Acad Med Sci Peking Union Med Coll 4:43–47
31. Zhang YC (1983) Epithelial dysplasia of the stomach and its relationship with gastric cancer. 6th Asia Pacific Cancer Conference, Sendai
32. Zhang YC, Sun ZX, Lin HZ, Zhang WF, Bai XW, Aoki K, Kawai K, Sasaki R, Tsuchihashi Y, Ito Y, Watanabe N (1987) Spectrum of gastric diseases in north China. In: Wada T, Aoki K, Yachi A (eds) Current status of cancer research in Asia, The Middle East and other countries. University of Nagoya Press, Nagoya, pp 41–49
33. Zhang YC, Zhang PF, Wang MX, Liu SQ (1988) Histopathologic types of gastric dysplasia. Chin J Cancer Res 1:47–52
34. Zhang YC, Lin HZ, Sun ZX, Bai XW, Aoki K, Kawai K, Sasaki R, Tsuchihashi Y, Ito Y, Watanabe Y (1989) Comparative etiologic study on gastric cancer in north China and north Japan. In: Sasaki R, Aoki K (eds) Epidemiology and prevention of cancer. University of Nagoya Press, Nagoya, pp 150–155

2 Precursors of Gastric Carcinoma*

P. Correa

Introduction

Two main histopathological types of gastric carcinoma have been identified, for which the names "intestinal" and "diffuse" have been coined [1]. The diffuse type is most frequently found in a mucosa which has a normal appearance outside the tumor. Although precancerous lesions have been described in some such cases, namely the "globoid dysplasia" [2] and the "nonmetaplastic dysplasia" [3], they are not found in most cases seen in general pathology practice.

Intestinal type tumors are surrounded by gastric mucosa showing chronic lesions which precede the carcinoma. These tumors are the subject of this chapter. Most intestinal type cancers make their appearance in a background of multifocal atrophic gastritis (MAG), whose sequelae include intestinal metaplasia and dysplasia [4]. MAG is the predominant type of chronic gastritis in countries whose inhabitants are at high risk from gastric cancer: Japan, China, Latin America, and Northern Europe. Another prominent form of atrophic gastritis, observed mostly in Scandinavian populations associated with the pernicious anemia syndrome, is diffuse corporal gastritis. Gastric cancer is also a late complication of gastrectomies, the so-called stump carcinoma. Very rare syndromes such as Ménétrier's gastritis, are occasionally seen as a background to gastric cancer. Gastric polyps may also give rise to carcinomas, especially the adenomatous polyps and less frequently the hyperplastic polyps.

Multifocal Chronic Atrophic Gastritis

It has been postulated that in the MAG syndrome a continuum of progressive changes precede clinical gastric carcinoma of the intestinal type. These changes are covered by the term "precursors" and fall into two basic

* Work supported by Grant No. P01-CA28842 from the National Cancer Institute.
Louisiana State University Medical Center, New Orleans, LA 70112, USA

Ying-Chan Zhang/Keiichi Kawai (Eds.)
Precancerous Conditions and Lesions of the Stomach

categories: those with mature and those with immature cellular phenotype. Lesions with a mature cellular phenotype are probably remote from the cancer end point, are highly prevalent in populations at high risk, and probably do not deserve any special surveillance or intervention by clinicians because most will never reach the stage of clinical cancer. Cells in precursor lesions with immature phenotype may have reached the stage of irreversibility to normal phenotype, represent a greater threat to the patient, and deserve close clinical surveillance.

The MAG complex can be subdivided into several components which appear to occur sequentially in time and are briefly described and illustrated below. All components are accompanied by interstitial infiltration of chronic inflammatory cells, mostly lymphocytes and plasma cells which are abundant in younger patients but tend to become scarce with age and when the other components of the MAG complex become more advanced. Another common lesion observed in most stages of the MAG spectrum is hyperplasia of the glandular necks, which seems to wax and wane in response to recent epithelial cell injury.

Atrophy

Gland loss in MAG occurs as multiple foci, more common around the antrum–corpus junction and the lesser curvature. The loss of glands leaves wide areas of the mucosa occupied by the stromal elements of the organ (Fig. 1). The antral glands appear as multiple sections of a coil, at least four of which should be observed in a section which represents the full thickness of the mucosa. Mild degrees of atrophy are difficult to document and are based on a decrease in the number of gland loops. Such glands may disappear entirely from extensive areas when the atrophy is severe.

Intestinal Metaplasia

Gastric glands lost in the process of atrophic gastritis are frequently replaced by cells with intestinal phenotypes. Metaplastic glands replace the closely packed tubular glands of the corporal and antral mucosa by crypt-like structures lined by absorptive and goblet cells typical of the intestinal mucosa. Argentaffin and Paneth cells are also present in some intestinalized crypts. Metaplastic glands can also occupy the foveolar region and surface epithelium, especially when this region is thicker than normal, an apparent result of previous foveolar hyperplasia. Structures resembling both small and large intestinal mucosa have been identified in metaplastic lesions of the gastric mucosa (Figs. 2, 3). Some observations suggest that in the initial stages of metaplasia the small intestinal type predominates, whereas in advanced lesions colonic type crypts are more frequent [5–8]. The two

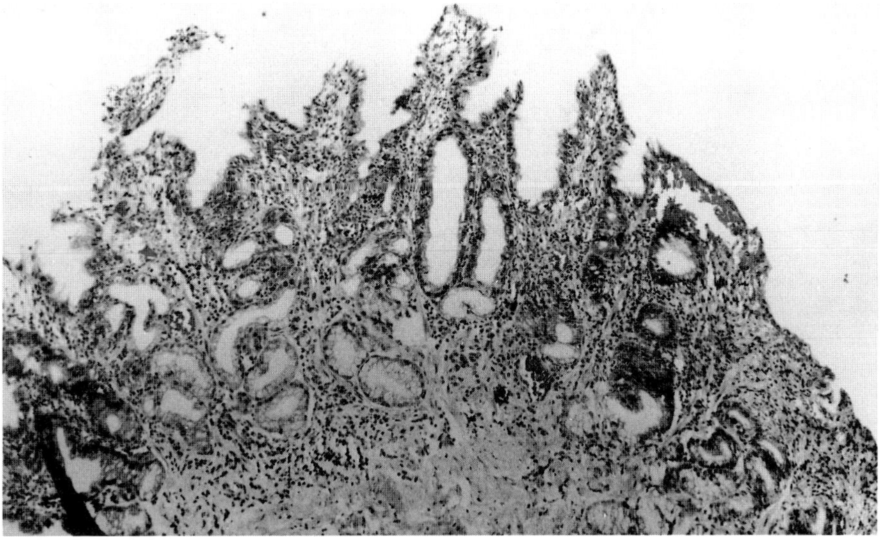

Fig. 1. Multifocal chronic atrophic gastritis (MAG). There is loss of antral glands, lymphocytic infiltrate, hyperplasia of gland necks, and depletion of mucin. Acute inflammation (activity) is superimposed on MAG

types often coexist, a situation that could be interpreted as a transition from small intestinal to colonic type. Cells of the small intestinal type of gastric metaplasia secrete the normal small intestinal sialomucin which stains with Alcian blue (pH 2.5) and does not take the high-iron diamine stain. The same cells usually secrete the complete set of intestinal enzymes: alkaline phosphatase, sucrase, leucine aminopeptidase, trehalase, succinic dehydrogenase, and diaphorase. For this reason, this type has been called "complete metaplasia" [9].

More advanced stages of the process often show the prominent colonic type of metaplasia, which has straight crypts lined by columnar cells with abundant cytoplasmic mucin, a brush border being absent (few microvilli). In this type of metaplastic mucosa, most small intestinal enzymes are absent, although sucrase and leucine aminopeptidase may persist in small amounts. For that reason, this metaplasia has been called "incomplete." The mucin secretion, a mixture of sialomucin and sulfated mucin, is typical of the large bowel; the latter stains positively with high-iron diamine. Several investigators, basing their reports on morphologic observations, have proposed that colonic metaplasia is more closely related to dysplasia and cancer than small intestinal metaplasia [5–8].

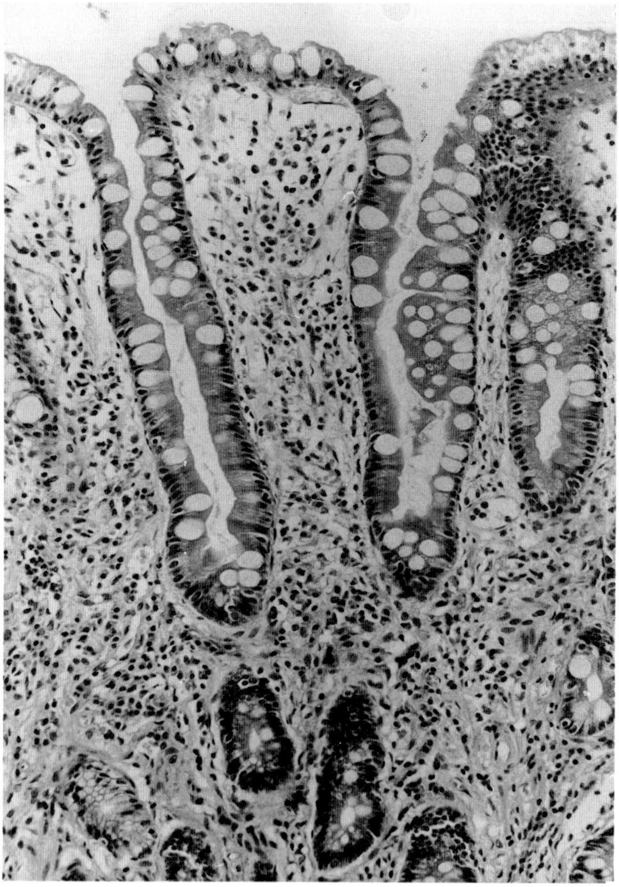

Fig. 2. Metaplasia of the small intestinal type. The surface is lined by absorptive cells with well formed brush border alternating with goblet cells

Dysplasia

The most frequent form of dysplasia in patients with MAG consists of proliferation of closely packed tubular glands which do not produce a gross elevation of the mucosa. This lesion has received the names "atypical epithelium" [10], "adenomatous dysplasia" [11] and "type I dysplasia" [12] (Fig. 4). The glands contain large, elongated, hyperchromatic nuclei which overlap one another in sections stained with hematoxylin and eosin. In mild dysplasias, the nuclei are mostly basal and elongated in shape. In moderate forms of dysplasia, the nuclei are closely packed, elongated, and pseudostratified, but retain some degree of polarity. In severe dysplasia, polarity is partially or totally lost, and the nuclei are oval or irregularly

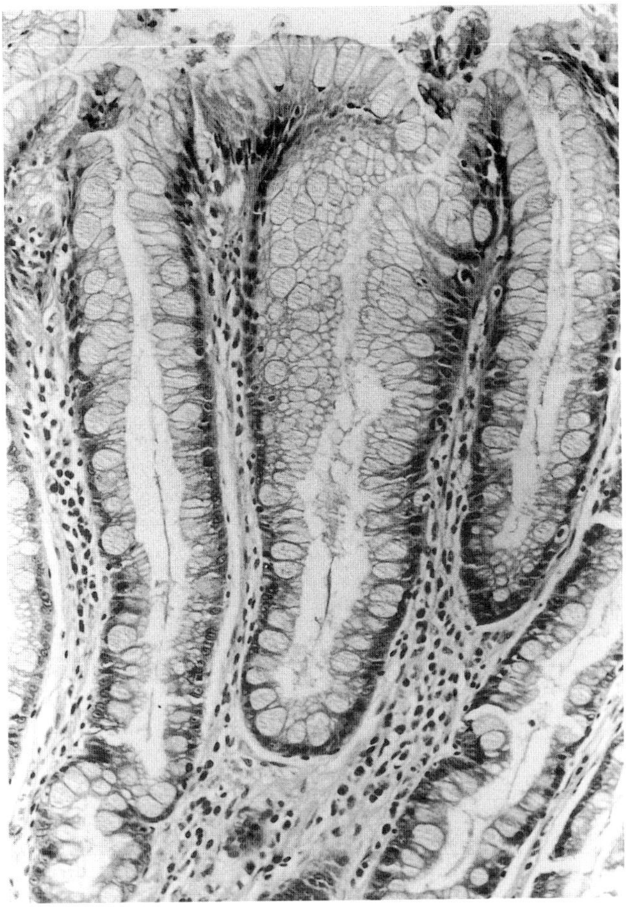

Fig. 3. Intestinal metaplasia, colonic type. Columnar cells with abundant mucin in small and large vacuoles line the lumen

shaped, have prominent nucleoli, show frequent mitosis, and often reach the top of the cell. Excessive proliferation of dysplastic glands results in the formation of a small mass which protrudes into the gastric lumen and constitutes an adenomatous polyp (Fig. 5). A less frequent form of dysplasia is the "hyperplastic" [11] or "type II" [12], in which the proliferating gland-like structures are irregularly shaped because of branching and formation of epithelial folds.

In mild forms of dysplasia, some absorptive cells with brush borders and goblet cells are well developed, and the nuclei are elongated but close to the basal side of the cell. In moderate dysplasias, some nuclei reach the upper part of the cell, show partial loss of polarity, and have moderately prominent nucleoli.

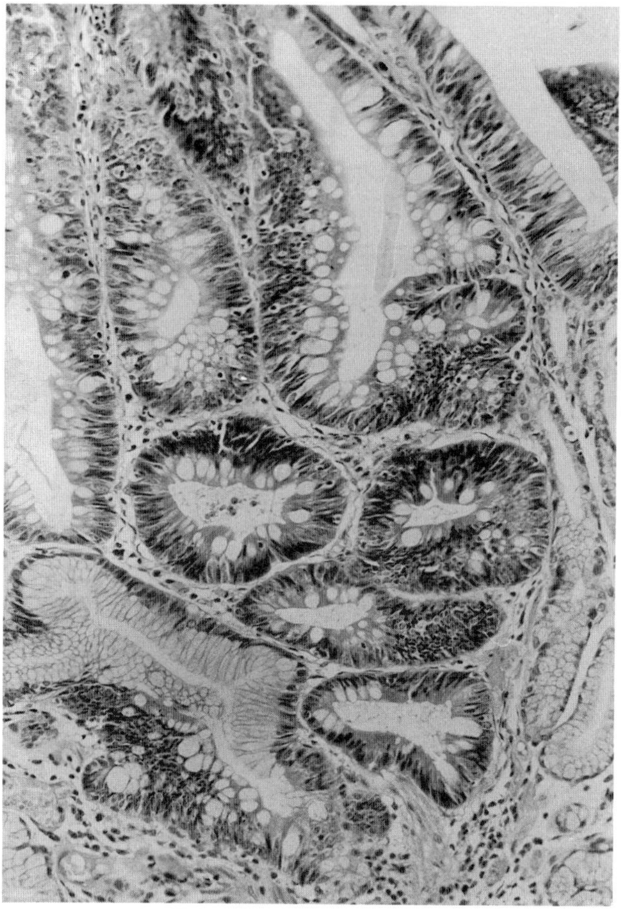

Fig. 4. Adenomatous dysplasia. Tubular glands line mucus-secreting cells with elongated, crowded, hyperchromatic nuclei

Severe dysplasias show the original glandular structures lined by cells with large, irregularly shaped nuclei with frequent mitosis, prominent nucleoli, and total loss of polarity. The transition from severe dysplasia to carcinoma-in-situ is difficult to define; the former usually shows neoplastic nuclei alternating with nuclei with lesser degrees of atypia.

Carcinomas arising in adenomatous dysplasia are usually well differentiated while those arising in hyperplastic dysplasias are of the intestinal type but poorly differentiated and spread laterally, partially replacing the foveolar epithelium. This corresponds to the so-called superficially spreading carcinoma.

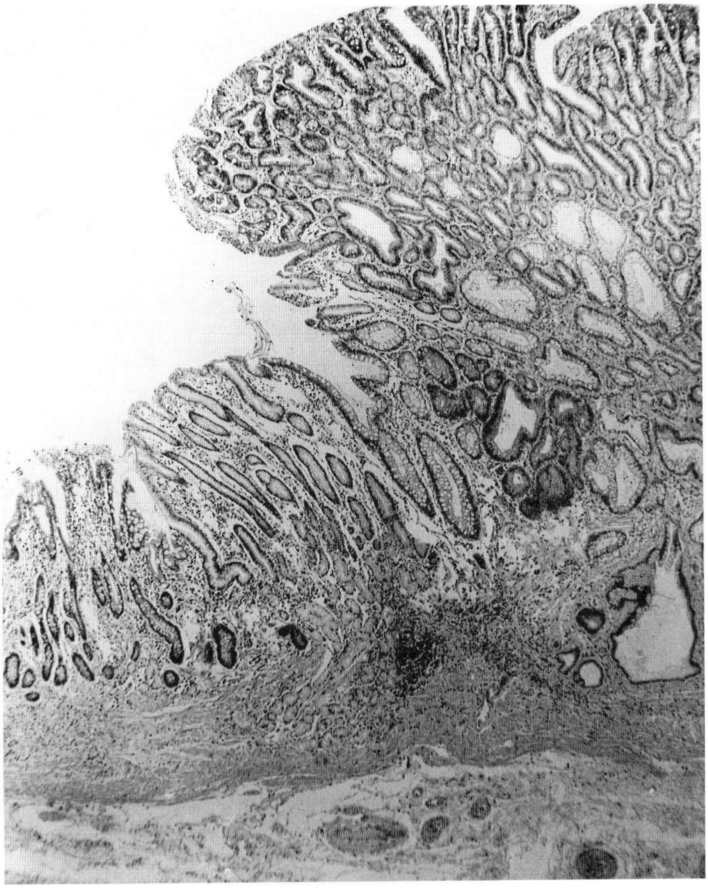

Fig. 5. Adenomatous polyp. Dysplastic tubular glands form the small mass of the polyp. Atrophic and metaplastic mucosae surround the polyp

Diffuse Corporal (Type A) Atrophic Gastritis

Diffuse corporal (type A) atrophic gastritis, a well characterized entity, is part of the pernicious anemia syndrome and characteristically appears in populations of Scandinavian extraction [13] (Fig. 6). It is for all practical purposes not seen in the areas of the world with the highest gastric cancer rates, such as Costa Rica, Japan, Chile and China. The lesion is frequently accompanied by high levels of gastrin and very low pepsinogen I levels in the blood, as well as high levels of parietal cell antibodies. The antrum may show superficial inflammation but is not atrophic. The oxyntic mucosa shows diffuse atrophy and extensive intestinal metaplasia.

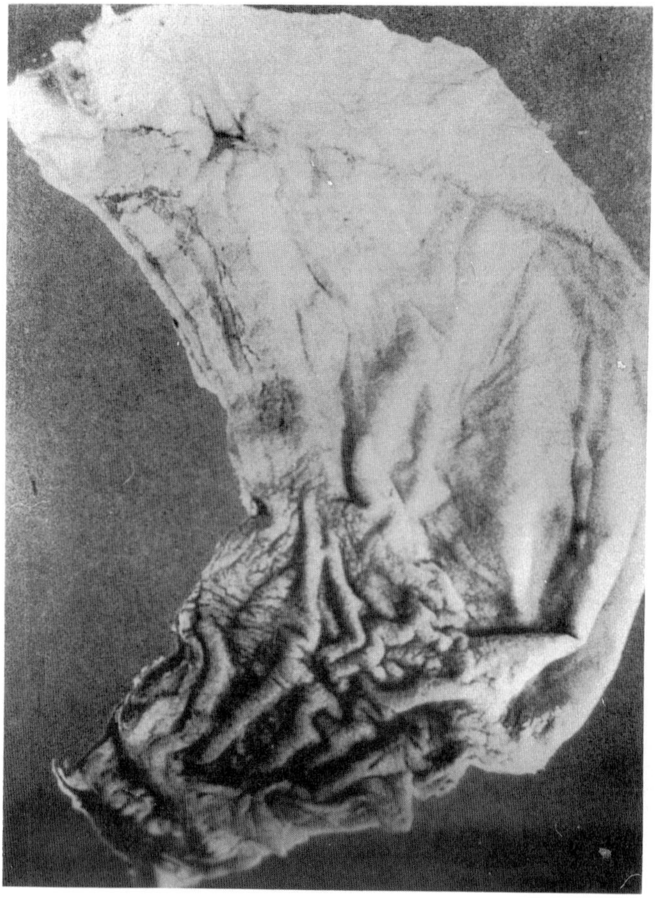

Fig. 6. Diffuse corporal (type A) gastritis. The antral mucosa is not atrophic but the oxyntic mucosa has lost the normal mucosal folds. (From [13])

Postgastrectomy Lesions

Several studies have shown that gastrectomy and gastroenteroanastomosis are predisposing factors for gastric carcinoma. This is especially true of operations which result in severe gastric reflux, such as the Billroth II technique. The gastric mucosa in such cases develops a characteristic type of inflammation known as "reflux gastritis," which is not known to give rise to precancerous lesions. The anastomotic site, however, is the frequent site of changes that may lead to invasive carcinoma. Such changes have been called "gastritis cystica polyposa" [14, 15] and have two histopathologic com-

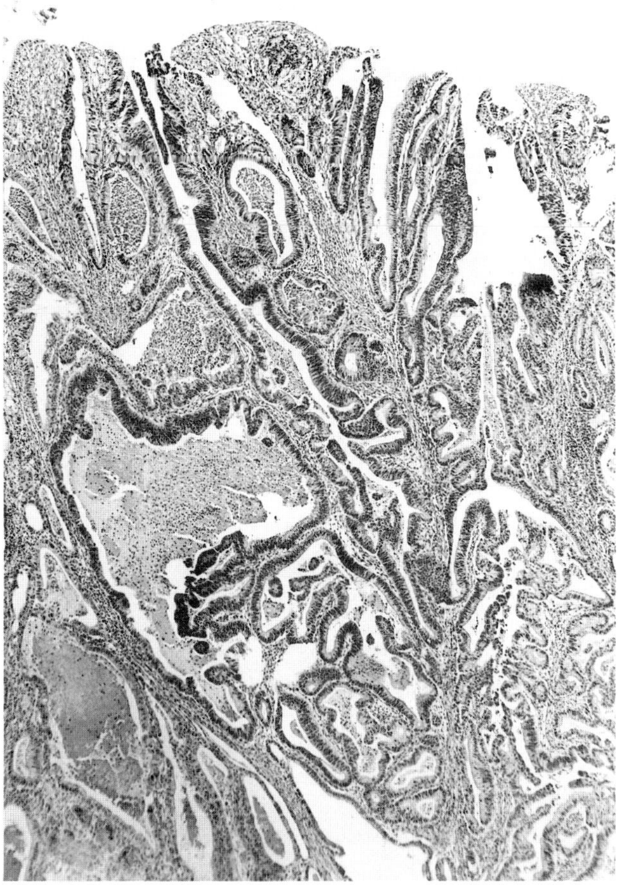

Fig. 7. Polyp from the gastroenteroanastomosis, previous Bilroth II gastrectomy. Markedly dysplastic villous and glandular structure. Gastritis cystica polyposa

ponents. The surface of the anastomosis becomes covered with a polyp of characteristic morphology. It is formed by multiple long villous structures lined by dysplastic epithelium (Fig. 7). It differs from the adenomatous polyps because it lacks the closely packed tubular glands. It differs from the hyperplastic polyp in that the epithelial cells do not have abundant mucin and the stroma is not edematous. At the base of the polyps small cysts are seen, again lined by dysplastic epithelium (Fig. 8). Such cysts penetrate the muscularis mucosa and the submucosa.

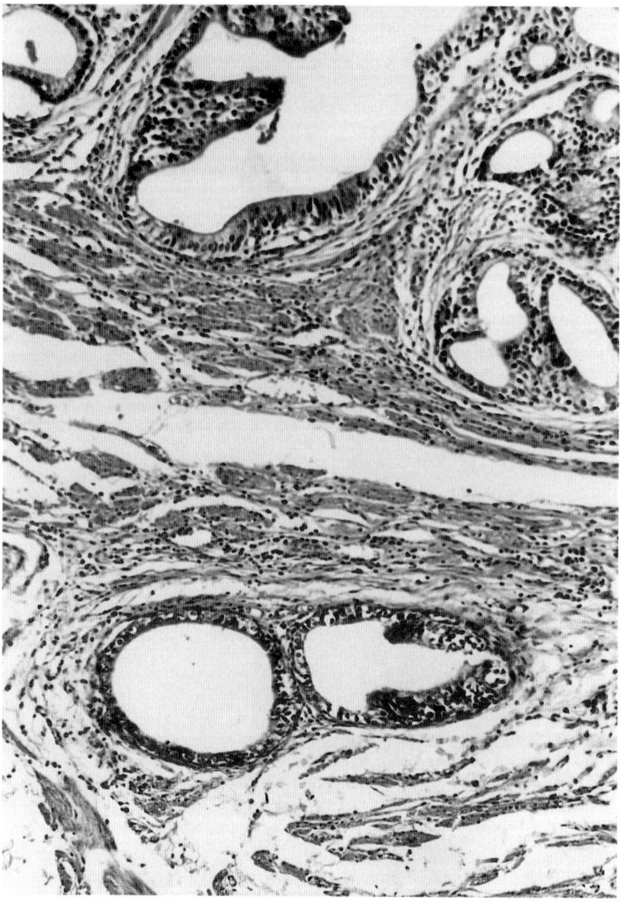

Fig. 8. Gastritis cystica polyposa (same specimen as that of Fig. 7). Cysts are lined by dysplastic cells penetrating the muscularis mucosae

Ménétrier's Disease

The characteristic lesion of the rare Ménétrier's disease is the elongation of the foveolar component of the gastric mucosa and the atrophy of the deep portion of the glands (Fig. 9). Cysts occasionally appear in the deep portion which are capable of penetrating the muscularis mucosa.

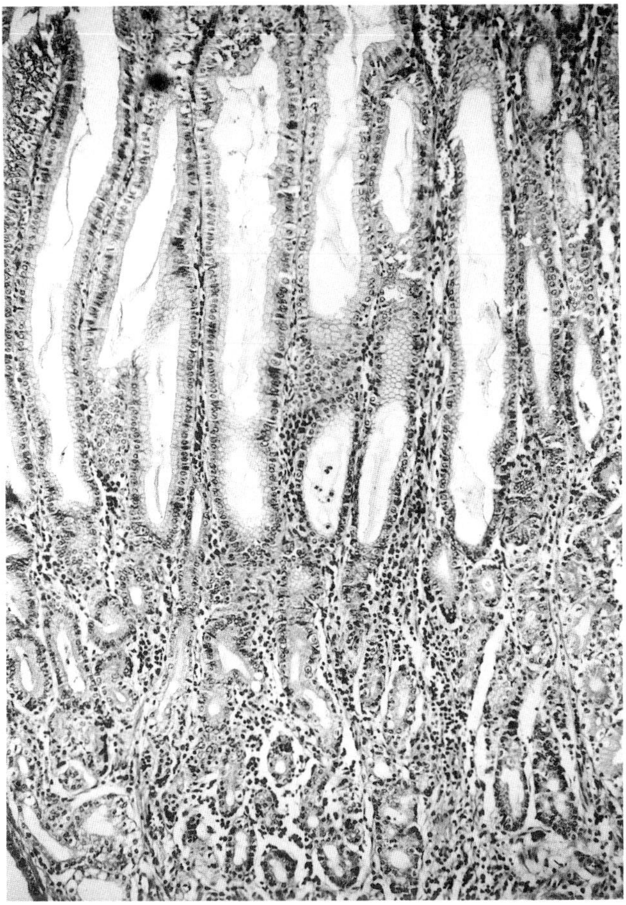

Fig. 9. Ménétrier's disease. Elongated and hyperplastic foveolae. Atrophic glands

Hyperplastic Polyps

These are exuberant proliferations of the foveolar components of the gastric glands which branch and acquire folds leading to star-shaped lumens. Characteristically the stroma is very edematous. Most polyps retain the above described morphology and because of this do not appear to give rise to carcinomas. Some hyperplastic polyps, especially those of a large size, may develop intestinal metaplasia and dysplastic adenomatous changes similar to those seen in MAG, and such morphologic background, appears potentially precancerous (Fig. 10).

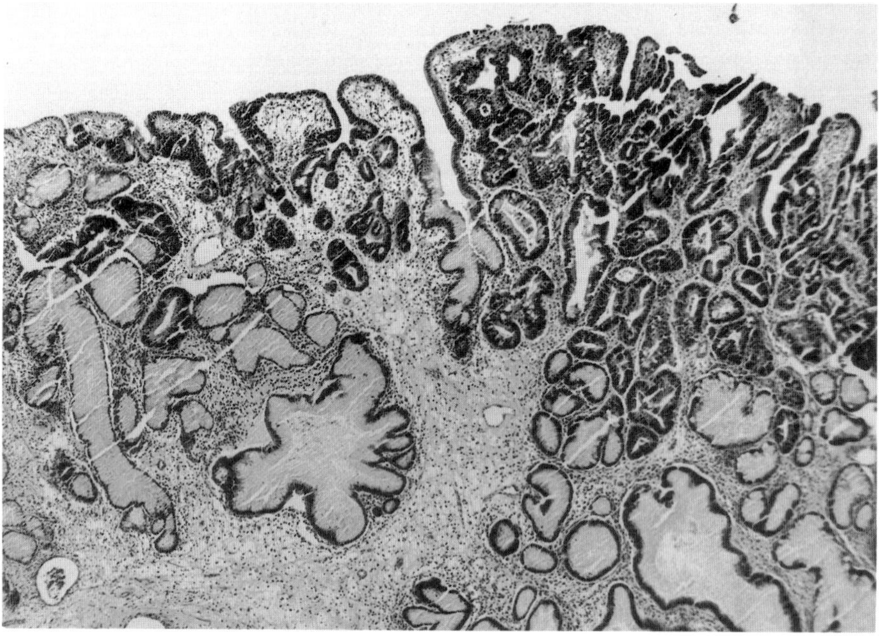

Fig. 10. Hyperplastic polyp showing the typical branching, mucus-rich, glands surrounded by edematous stroma. *Upper right*: adenomatous dysplasia and intestinal metaplasia

References

1. Lauren P (1965) The two histological main types of gastric carcinoma: diffuse and so-called intestinal-type carcinoma: an attempt at a histoclinical classification. Acta Pathol Microbiol Scand 64:31–49
2. Borchard F, Mittelstaedt A, Stux G (1979) Dysplasien im Resektionsmagen und Klassifikationsprobleme verschiedener Dysplasieformen. Verh Dtsch Ges Pathol 63: 250–257
3. Gandhur-Mnaymneh L, Paz J, Roldan E, Cassay J (1988) Dysplasia in non-metaplastic gastric mucosa. Am J Clin Pathol 12:96–114
4. Correa P (1988) A human model of gastric carcinogenesis. Cancer Res 48:3554–3560
5. Heilman KL, Hopker WW (1979) Loss of differentiation in intestinal metaplasia in cancerous stomachs. A comprehensive morphologic study. Pathol Res Pract 164: 249–258
6. Jass JR, Filipe MI (1979) Variants of intestinal metaplasia associated with gastric carcinoma. Histopathology 3:191–199
7. Sipponen P, Seppala K, Varis K, Hjelt L, Ihamaki T, Kekki M, Siurala M (1981) Intestinal metaplasia with colonic type sulfomucins: its association with gastric carcinoma. Acta Pathol Microbiol Scand 88:217–224
8. Teglbjaerg S, Nielsen HO (1978) Small intestinal type and colonic type intestinal metaplasia of the human stomach. Acta Pathol Microbiol Scand 86:351–355
9. Matsukura N, Susuki K, Kawachi T, Aoyagi M, Sugimura T, Kitaoka H, Numajiri H, Shirota A, Itahashi M, Hirota T (1980) Distribution of marker enzymes and mucin in

intestinal metaplasia in human stomachs and relation of complete and incomplete types of intestinal metaplasia to minute gastric carcinomas. JNCI 65:231–240
10. Sugano H, Kyoichi N, Takagi K (1972) An atypical epithelium of the stomach. A clinico-pathological entity. Gann Monogr Cancer Res 11:257–269
11. Cuello C, Correa P, Zarama G, Lopez J, Murray J, Gordillo G (1979) Histopathology of gastric dysplasias: correlations with gastric juice chemistry. Am J Surg Pathol 3:491–500
12. Jass JR (1983) A classification of gastric dysplasias. Histopathology 7:181–193
13. Strickland RG, McKay IR (1973) A reappraisal of the nature and significance of chronic atrophic gastritis. Dig Dis 18:426–446
14. Littler ER, Gleiberman NE (1972) Gastritis cystica polyposa. Cancer 29:205–209
15. Appelman HD (1984) Localized and extensive expansions of the gastric mucosa: mucosal polyps and giant folds. In: Appelman HD (ed) Pathology of the esophagus, stomach and duodenum. Churchill Livingstone, New York, pp 79–119

3 An Epidemiological Study of the Ratio of Gastric Ulcer to Duodenal Ulcer: Its Relationship to Gastric Cancer

K. Kawai, Y. Watanabe, and K. Hayashi

Introduction

We have previously reported that atrophic gastritis and intestinal metaplasia of the gastric mucosa, which are both regarded as precancerous conditions of gastric cancer, have similar etiologies [1]. Atrophic change of gastric mucosa was found in a few Japanese patients with duodenal ulcer [2], and the localization of peptic ulcers in the stomach correlated with the extent of coexisting atrophic gastritis [3]. With ulcers of the antrum, closed type 1 gastric mucosal atrophy was seen most frequently, and the antral mucosa became broader with development of peptic ulcers at more proximal sites of the stomach [2]. In the countries where gastric ulcer patients are more frequent than duodenal ulcer patients, the mortality rate from gastric cancer apppears to be high. We therefore consider that the gastric ulcer to duodenal ulcer ratio (GU/DU) is an indicator of possible gastric cancer development.

In this chapter, we examine GU/DU as a marker of coexisting atrophic gastritis with respect to its relationship to gastric cancer, and possible nutritional factors related to the development of gastric cancer.

GU/DU as a Marker of Coexistent Gastritis in the Japanese Population

In Japan, among those suffering from peptic ulcer, deaths caused by gastric ulcer and duodenal ulcer have been reported separately. The mortality rates from these ulcers have been decreasing in both sexes for the last 30 years, and gastric to duodenal ulcer mortality ratios have shown an overall decrease for both men and women [4].

Figure 1 shows the trends in Japan of sex-age standardized mortality rates from gastric ulcer and gastric cancer, standardized mortality ratios

Department of Preventive Medicine, Kyoto Prefectural University of Medicine, Kawaramachi Hirokoji, Kamikyoku, Kyoto, Japan

Ying-Chan Zhang/Keiichi Kawai (Eds.)
Precancerous Conditions and Lesions of the Stomach

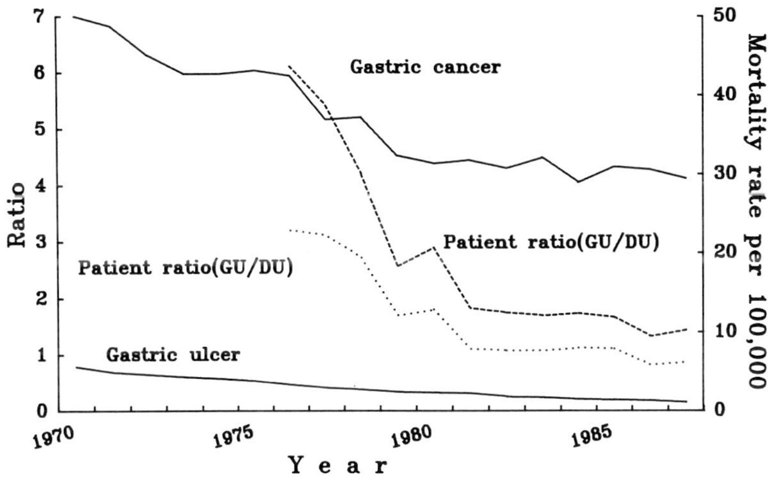

Fig. 1. Trends in gastric ulcer to duodenal ulcer ratio (GU/DU) and mortality from gastric diseases in Japan

(gastric ulcer to duodenal ulcer, GU/DU), and crude ratios of gastric to duodenal ulcer patients (GU/DU) and of gastric to duodenal and gastric ulcer patients (GU/GU + DU) confirmed by endoscopy at our university hospital from 1976. The GU/DU mortality ratio corresponds to the clinical GU/DU patient ratio during this period. Both the adjusted Japanese mortality from gastric cancer and the patient GU/DU ratio in the hospitals have shown a similar decline at an almost constant rate.

We are able to diagnose atrophic gastritis radiographically or endoscopically. The required information can be taken from the prevalence rate or incidence rate of atrophic gastric mucosa among the population as a possible precancerous condition, although we have no mortality statistics or clinical statistics for atrophic gastritis.

There is some clinical evidence that the incidence of duodenal ulcer has been increasing over the past 30 years, as demonstrated radiographically or endoscopically. However, the ratio of gastric ulcer to duodenal ulcer has been decreasing during this period.

We are able to explain this change in GU/DU ratio from clinical statistics as well as from mortality statistics. Indeed, from our analysis, the mortality statistics (Fig. 1) are in agreement with the clinical statistics with respect to the GU/DU ratio. These findings suggest that GU/DU ratio, calculated from mortality statistics, can reflect the state of the gastric mucosae of the population. Atrophic gastritis is a variable condition which may have a predisposition to gastric cancer.

GU/DU in Prefectures in Japan

In the Japanese population, there is a tendency for gastric mucosae to develop gastric ulcers, and a background of atrophic gastritis is an important factor in the etiology of gastric cancer. We now present a clinical review of GU/DU in prefectures in Japan.

As previously reported [5], we randomly selected one public hospital per prefecture from a 1984 list of hospitals in Japan designated for residency or authorized by the Japanese Society of Gastroendoscopy. We recorded the age and sex of all peptic ulcer patients with gastric or duodenal ulcer (including those with ulcer scarring) endoscopically diagnosed during 1984.

When a hospital declined to take part in the study, a second hospital was randomly chosen. If a third hospital declined, the prefecture was excluded from the study. We selected two hospitals from both Hokkaido and Tokyo, because of their large populations. For Okinawa, original data compiled by the Okinawa Gastroenterologists' Association was used, which included all peptic ulcers investigated in 45 medical institutes in Okinawa from 1982 to 1983 [6]. The crude GU/DU ratio was determined for each prefecture.

Table 1 shows the crude GU/DUs for each prefecture. The crude GU/DU ratio for Hokkaido was 3:1 or above, indicating a high incidence of gastric ulcer. The GU/DU was less than 1:1 for Okinawa prefecture, indicating a high incidence of duodenal ulcer. In most areas, the ratio was between 1:1 and 2:1 indicating a slightly higher incidence of gastric ulcer. These results demonstrate clear regional differences.

The downward trend of the adjusted mortality rate for gastric cancer was demonstrated, and the declining GU/DU mentioned previously suggests that GU/DU is a possible indicator of development of gastric cancer. The prefectural comparisons of GU/DU demonstrated a remarkable contrast between Hokkaido and Okinawa. However, it is doubtful whether data from one or several hospitals can accurately reflect the characteristics of the region, so the possibility of a selection bias cannot be excluded.

GU/DU in Asian Countries

The GU/DUs of prefectures in Japan showed regional differences: the value of GU/DU for most parts of Honshu, Shikoku, and Kyushu are between 1:1 and 2:1; for Hokkaido, more than 3:1, and for Okinawa where the mortality from gastric cancer is lowest in Japan, less than 1:1. We will attempt to clarify the GU/DU ratio in Asian countries neighboring Japan.

Using the same procedure as that employed in the previous investigation in Japan, we recorded the age and sex of all patients with gastric or

Table 1. Crude ratio of gastric ulcer to duodenal ulcer (GU/DU) in prefectures in Japan in 1984

Prefecture	Male	Female	Total
Hokkaido	3.25	4.28	3.51
Aomori	2.19	2.10	2.17
Iwate	1.05	0.89	1.00
Yamagata	1.55	1.52	1.54
Tochigi	1.18	1.35	1.23
Gunma	1.42	1.06	1.29
Saitama	1.27	1.23	1.26
Chiba	1.38	1.29	1.36
Tokyo	2.16	2.50	2.24
Kanagawa	1.02	0.71	0.93
Niigata	1.70	1.43	1.62
Toyama	2.18	2.35	2.22
Ishikawa	1.76	1.75	1.76
Hukui	1.46	1.35	1.43
Nagano	1.31	1.59	1.37
Gihu	1.49	1.35	1.45
Shizuoka	1.45	1.53	1.47
Shiga	1.74	1.54	1.32
Kyoto	2.43	2.89	2.53
Osaka	2.84	4.47	3.18
Hyougo	1.44	1.32	1.41
Nara	1.79	2.56	1.95
Wakayama	1.61	1.85	1.68
Shimane	1.89	2.14	1.95
Okayama	2.43	2.62	2.48
Hiroshima	1.44	2.21	1.60
Yamaguchi	1.42	1.19	1.34
Kagawa	1.51	1.25	1.44
Kochi	2.60	2.41	2.55
Hukuoka	1.05	1.45	1.15
Nagasaki	2.12	1.82	2.04
Kumamoto	1.88	1.32	1.63
Oita	2.31	1.52	2.04
Miyazaki	2.16	1.57	2.00
Kagoshima	1.30	1.25	1.28
Okinawa[a]	0.89	0.93	0.90

[a] 1982–1983

duodenal ulcer (including those with ulcer scarring) endoscopically diagnosed during 1984 at designated hospitals in Korea, China, Taiwan, Hong Kong, the Philippines, and Thailand. The doctors participating in the study were physicians or surgeons who specialized in gastroendoscopy. We used 1980 data in several hospitals. As the standard population, we adopted the Japanese peptic ulcer patients (21622) reported in our previous investigation [4]. The male, female, and total GU/DU ratios were adjusted by this standard population.

Table 2. Age-standardized ratio of gastric ulcer to duodenal ulcer (GU/DU) in Asian countries in 1984

Country	Number of GU and DU cases	Age-standardized GU/DU		
		Male	Female	Total
Japan[a]	21 622	1.66	1.65	1.66
Korea				
Seoul	642	0.79	0.52	0.64
Kwangju[b]	285	2.70	4.32	3.03
China				
Beijing[b]	479	0.73	0.65	0.72
X' ian[b]	217	0.91	0.74	0.86
Sining	161	2.02	1.63	1.91
Shenyang	275	1.30	0.99	1.22
Guangzhou	658	0.26	0.23	0.25
Taiwan	11 317	0.52	0.49	0.51
Taibei	7 810	0.53	0.48	0.52
Taizong	2 677	0.54	0.10	0.39
Tainan	832	0.42	0.43	0.42
Hong Kong	333	0.59	0.67	0.63
Philippines				
Manila	319	1.19	1.76	1.36
Thailand				
Bangkok	85	3.13	2.42	2.74

[a] Except Okinawa
[b] In 1980

Table 2 shows the revised GU/DUs of hospitals according to city and country (district) where the research was conducted. In Korea, whose altitude is the same as that of Japan, the ratio was less than 1:1 in Seoul, but more than 1:1 in Kwangju. The ratio in each area of Taiwan, and also in Hong Kong, was less than 1:1, while in the Philippines and Thailand it was more than 1:1. In China, different hospitals showed different GU/DUs: less than 1:1 for Beijing, X'ian and Guangzhou, and more than 1:1 for Shenyang and Sining. Regional differences were evident.

These data are all from endoscopic findings with a high degree of accuracy, however it should not be concluded that these differences are due to regional and/or ethnic differences, because data complied from only one hospital were used for each region. Therefore, the location of the hospital and the socioeconomic background of local people may have generated the special characteristics of the region, expressed as the different GU/DUs observed in the same country. It is more appropriate to regard the differences as reflecting different characteristics of studied population, rather than the characteristics of each country.

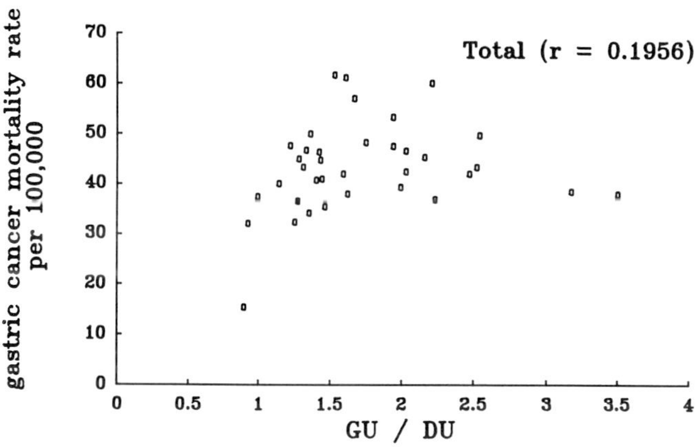

Fig. 2. Correlation between gastric ulcer to duodenal ulcer (GU/DU) and gastric cancer mortality rates for prefectures in Japan

GU/DU and Gastric Cancer Mortality

The recent downward trend in revised mortality rate for gastric cancer in Japan coincides with the narrowing of the GU/DU observed clinically in hospitals. From this finding, we previously reported that the GU/DU in a certain population may be an indicator of gastric cancer [3]. We therefore reviewed the correlation between GU/DU and mortality from gastric cancer, in prefectures in Japan and districts in other Asian countries.

Correlation between GU/DU and Gastric Cancer Mortality Among Prefectures in Japan

A correlative diagram and Pearson's correlation coefficient were obtained and tested with respect to the relation between the crude GU/DUs in 1984 (see "GU/DU in Prefectures in Japan", p. 23) and the crude mortality from gastric cancer in 1985 [7].

Figure 2 shows the correlation between the crude GU/DU (1984), which is a combined ratio of both males and females for 36 prefectures including Tokyo, and the crude mortality rate for gastric cancer (1985) [8]. The coefficient of correlation is 0.1956, and there was no statistical significance. If this analysis is conducted according to sex, then $r = 0.2180$ in males and $r = 0.1403$ in females; these figures are not statistically significant [8].

Although the method of analysis of the Patient Survey [9] using random sampling conducted by the Japanese Ministry of Health and Welfare is ideal, this survey used combined statistical figures of gastric ulcer and duodenal ulcer. Data from endoscopic examinations with a high accuracy were used for our study. If the extrapolated selection bias is small, then a study focusing on two regions, Hokkaido and Okinawa, illustrating the extreme values of GU/DU, may be able to elucidate the correlation between GU/DU and gastric cancer. However, our analysis did not confirm a statistically significant correlation.

The correlation between these two indicators cannot be proven or disproven for the following reasons:

1. Both are cross-sectional data, and the 1-year interval between the two data poses a problem for the temporal relationship of association.
2. The mortality rate from gastric cancer does not necessarily reflect the morbidity rate for gastric cancer in 1985.
3. The peptic ulcer data from one or two hospitals may not represent the actual state of peptic ulcers in the prefecture.

If the prefectures with the highest GU/DUs, Hokkaido and Osaka, are excluded from the analysis, the correlation coefficient is higher (0.3952, $p < 0.05$). No statistically significant correlation was established in the analysis. However, the validity of the analytical method employed is uncertain, and further research on the correlation between GU/DU and gastric cancer is required.

Correlation between GU/DU and Gastric Cancer Mortality Among Asian Countries

We collected data on the mortality from gastric cancer in 1984, according to sex and age in each country [10–13], which was standardized with world cancer mortality statistics given by Segi [14] to obtain the adjusted mortality. When 1984 data were not available, we used the data of the nearest year. In China, we used 1973–1975 data [15], which are already adjusted by the same standard population [14]. If no appropriate data were available, we did not include it in the analysis.

Table 3 shows the revised mortality rate for gastric cancer in Asian countries (in many countries, the calculation was not conducted in 1984). The mortality rates were high (>20 per 100 000 population) in Japan and Korea, and also in the Chinese provinces of Shaanxi, Qinghai, and Liaoning (whose major city is Shenyang). The rates in Taiwan, Hong Kong and the Chinese province of Guangdong were moderate, (approximately ten per 100 000 population). In the Philippines and Thailand they were low (<ten per 100 000 population).

Comparisons of the mortality rates from gastric cancer in different countries must be considered. In countries where the prevalence of gastric ulcer is greater than that of duodenal ulcer, with a GU/DU of 1:1 and over, mortality rates for gastric cancer are high. However, in countries such as Taiwan and Hong Kong, where duodenal ulcers outnumber gastric ulcers, GU/DUs being less than 1:1, the mortality rates for gastric cancer are low.

Table 3. Age-standardized mortality rate from gastric cancer in Asian countries

Country	Year	Mortality rate[a] from gastric cancer		
		Male	Female	Total
Japan	1984	42.7	20.2	29.9
Korea	1985	57.3	25.1	38.7
China				
Beijing	1973	22.3	10.5	–
Shaanxi		36.5	20.4	–
Qinghai	~	79.5	42.2	–
Liaoning		45.8	20.7	–
Guangdong	1975	11.4	5.1	–
Taiwan	1988	16.1	8.2	12.4
Hongkong	1984	11.1	5.4	8.1
Philippines	1977	6.2	4.9	5.6
Thailand	1981	1.9	0.9	1.3

–, no data
[a] Per 100 000 population

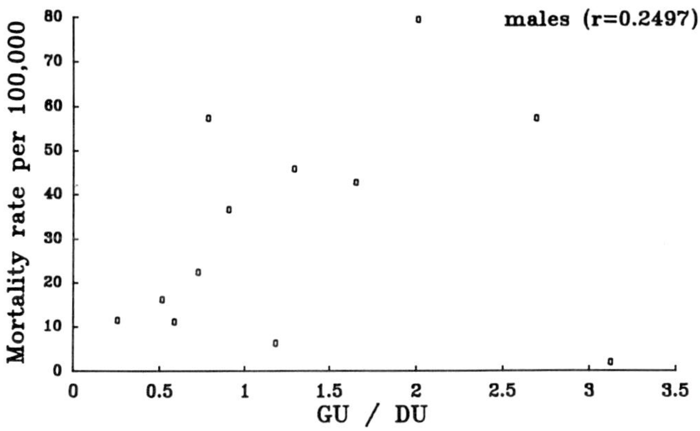

Fig. 3. Correlation between gastric ulcer to duodenal ulcer (GU/DU) and gastric cancer mortality rate in males in Asian countries

These data of gastric death rates and GU/DU (see "GU/DU in Asian Countries", p. 24) were used to construct and test a correlative diagram and Pearson's correlation coefficient.

Figure 3 shows the correlation between the age-adjusted mortality rate from gastric cancer in males, and the sex- and age-adjusted GU/DUs of 12 hospitals (districts) [16]. In males and females, respectively, $r = 0.2497$ and 0.2177 [16]. These figures are small and have no statistical significance. This may be because direct comparisons of the mortality statistics of a country with the statistics of one hospital are not justifiable. It is possible that a disproportionately high percentage of patients who consulted a surveyed hospital belong to either the high or low income bracket. Furthermore, the gastric cancer mortality rate does not necessarily represent the incidence of gastric cancer. One possible hypothesis is that the regions where duodenal ulcers outnumber gastric ulcers, (GU/DU being less than 1:1), are economically affluent, and the incidence of gastric cancer is low.

If the data of Kwangju and Bangkok are excluded from the analysis, the correlation coefficients are increased (male:0.7128 ($p < 0.01$), female:0.3935) [16]. Further investigation of the possibility of correlation between GU/DU and the gastric cancer mortality rate is required.

Gastric Cancer and Nutrition

We have reported in a separate study that in Japan protein possibly protects people from peptic ulcer disease [4]. The aim of this section is to determine the correlation between gastric cancer mortality [17] and nutrition, including protein consumption, in Japanese society [18]. We also review nutrition with respect to its possible relation to gastric cancer occurrence.

To review the significance of nutrition, i.e., calorie, protein, fat, and oil consumption, in relation to gastric cancer mortality, we conducted multiple regression analysis, using statistics relating to daily per capita consumption of the Japanese population from 1970 to 1981.

Table 4 shows the results of multiple regression analysis of the changes in gastric cancer and nutrition. In both sexes, the partial regression coefficients are positive for energy, and negative for both protein and oil and fat. The absolute value of the partial regression coefficient is approximately 0.5 for both sexes.

We performed multiple regression analysis of changes in gastric cancer and changes in nutrition induced by economic growth. The results of our

Table 4. Multiple regression analysis between gastric cancer mortality rate and food consumption[a] in Japan

Items	Coefficient of gastric cancer mortality rate	
	Male	Female
Calorie	0.0143	0.0069
Protein	−0.4015	−0.2068
Oil and fat	−0.1119	−0.0546
Multiple regression coefficient (square)	0.5053	0.4813

[a] Five-year period prior to gastric cancer mortality

analyses indicates that protein is most closely related to mortality associated with gastric cancer; high protein consumption tends to be associated with a lower rate of gastric cancer.

The result of this analysis is not the standardized partial regression coefficient. However, the absolute value can be regarded as the level of relation that each factor has for changes of gastric cancers, since it is calculated as the ratio of the explanatory variate to the 1970 value. Consequently, the hypothesis that the decreasing mortality rate is associated with high protein consumption in the affluent economical background of Japan is possible.

However, in addition to this hypothesis (a district with a GU/DU of less than 1:1 and a higher incidence of duodenal ulcer is affluent), a second possible hypothesis (in Japan, with its increasingly affluent society, gastric cancer mortality rates have been decreasing with increased protein consumption) is also logical. Further analysis of factors relating to regional differences in GU/DU ratios, and the correlation between GU/DUs and gastric cancer, are required by direct epidemiological analysis of human subjects.

References

1. Hayashi K, Watanabe Y, Uozumi G, Inokuchi H, Misaki F, Kohli M, Kato T, Okuda J, Miura H, Ida K, Kawai K (1985) An epidemiological study on intestinal metaplasia of stomach (in Japanese). J Kyoto Prefect Univ Med 9:883–888
2. Kawai K, Yamaguchi K, Fujimoto S, Misaki F (1980) The features of peptic ulcer in Japan. In: Huang Ming-Xin (ed) Proceedings of International Cimetidines Symposium, Shanghai 1980. Shanghai Scientific and Technological Literature, Shanghai, pp 114–123
3. Kawai K, Aoike A, Hayashi K, Liu HH, Watanabe Y (1990) Is atrophic gastritis or intestinal metaplasia precancerous condition of gastric cancer? Nagoya University Press, Nagoya, pp 144–149
4. Kawai K, Shirakawa K, Misaki F, Hayashi K, Watanabe Y (1989) Natural history and epidemiologic studies of peptic ulcer disease in Japan. Gastroenterology 96:581–585
5. Kawai K, Watanabe Y (1987) Epidemiological aspect of peptic ulcers in Japan. In: Oda T (ed) New trends in peptic ulcer and chronic hepatitis, part 1. Peptic ulcer. Excerpta Medica, Amsterdam, pp 3–9
6. Miura T, Shimabukuro T, Sakumoto K, Kinjo F, Kawashima M, Keida Y, Takazato Y, Yamauchi Y, Maeda K (1987) Features of peptic ulcer in Okinawa. In: Oda T (ed) New trends in peptic ulcer and chronic hepatitis, part 1. Peptic ulcer. Excerpta Medica, Amsterdam, pp 10–14
7. Statistic and Information Department of Ministry of Health and Welfare (1988) Standardized mortality rate from main cause in 1985. Health and Welfare Association, Tokyo
8. Watanabe Y, Hayashi K, Saito A, Kawai K (1990) A cross-sectional study on gastric cancer death and gastric ulcer to duodenal ulcer ratio in Japan (in Japanese). J Kyoto Prefect Univ Med 99:1305–1308
9. Statistic and Information Department of Ministry of Health and Welfare (1986) Patient Survey. Health and Welfare Association, Tokyo

10. World Health Organization (1986) World health statistics annual 1986. WHO, Geneva
11. World Health Organization (1987) World health statistics annual 1987. WHO, Geneva
12. World Health Organization (1988) World health statistics annual 1988. WHO, Geneva
13. Department of Health Executive Yuan, Taiwan Provincial Health Department, Taipei City Health Department and Kaohsiung City Health Department (1989) Health statistics 2: Vital statistics 1988. Republic of China
14. Segi M, Aoki K, Kurihara M (1981) World cancer mortality. Cancer mortality and morbidity statistics Japan and the world. Gann Monogr Cancer Res 26:121–123
15. Editorial Committee (1981) Atlas of cancer mortality in the People's Republic of China. China Map Press, Beijing
16. Watanabe Y, Saito A, Liu HH, Hayashi K, Kawai K (1990) An epidemiological study on gastric ulcer to duodenal ulcer ratio and gastric cancer death in Asian country (in Japanese). J Kyoto Prefect Univ Med 100:159–163
17. Statistics and Information Department of Ministry of Health and Welfare (1983) Vital statistics 1970–1981. Society of Health and Welfare Statistics, Tokyo
18. Research Division of Ministry of Agriculture and Forestry (1983) List of food demand/supply 1981. Society of Agriculture and Forestry Statistics, Tokyo

4 Gastric Polyps and Gastric Carcinoma

S.-C. Ming

Introduction

Definition

Polyps are nodular lesions which project above the mucosal surface. Depending on the location of the bulk of the lesion the polyps can be divided into intraluminal and intramural types. The latter is usually produced by a submucosal lesion whereas the former is a mucosal lesion. We are concerned here with the intraluminal polyp in terms of its relationship with gastric carcinoma. This kind of polyp has prominent epithelial components in which malignant transformation may occur. The mucosae surrounding such lesions are often abnormal and may also become the site of carcinoma development.

Incidence

Gastric polyps are not common, occurring in about 0.4% of the general adult population, as evidenced by autopsy or radiological survey [25]. Among clinical cases they account for about 3% of all gastric tumors and 41% of all benign gastric tumors [24]. Among endoscopy patients the incidence is 3%–5% [22, 37] and they account for 90% of benign tumors. Fifty percent of polyps occur in the antrum. Approximately 85% of them are less than 2 cm in diameter. About 80% of gastric polyp patients are over 50 years of age.

In patients with diseased stomach the incidence of polyps is much higher: 22%–37% in patients with pernicious anemia [7, 42], 6% in patients with chronic atrophic gastritis [39], and 4%–20% in the gastric remnants of partial gastrectomy [15, 36]. Carcinomas are commonly found in stomachs containing polyps. In one study, 44% of consecutively resected carcinomatous stomachs had polyps [28].

Department of Pathology, Temple University School of Medicine, Philadelphia, PA 19140, USA

Ying-Chan Zhang/Keiichi Kawai (Eds.)
Precancerous Conditions and Lesions of the Stomach

Table 1. Classification of benign epithelial gastric polyps

Neoplastic polyp: adenoma
Flat (tubular) adenoma: elevated or depressed
Papillary (villous) adenoma
Nonneoplastic polyp
Hyperplastic polyp
Hamartomatous polyp: with polyposis or isolated
Peutz-Jeghers polyp
Juvenile polyp
Fundic gland polyp
Inflammatory polyp
Inflammatory (retention) polyp
Polyp in Cronkhite-Canada syndrome
Heterotopic polyp
Ectopic pancreatic tissue
Ectopic Brunner gland hyperplasia

Classification and Pathology

The diagnosis of gastric polyp is based on the histological features of the lesion. In general the polyps are composed of glands and supporting stromal tissue. The architectural arrangements as well as the cytological features are used for definitive diagnosis. Based on these features epithelial gastric polyps can be classified into two major types: (a) the neoplastic type, and (b) the nonneoplastic type (Table 1). The distinction between these two types is based primarily on the cytological characteristics of the epithelial cells. Neoplastic polyps are composed of immature dysplastic epithelial cells whereas nonneoplastic polyps are composed of normal-appearing or regenerative epithelial cells.

Neoplastic Polyp

Neoplastic polyps are adenomas. They can be further divided according to the gross morphology of the lesion into flat and papillary types. The flat adenoma has a flat, although slightly irregular, mucosal surface whereas the papillary adenoma has a nodular surface with papillary lobulation. Adenomas are not common, accounting for only about 10% of polyps in the stomach in most reports [22, 31, 40], although an incidence as high as 25% has also been reported [44]. The incidence increases with age, with an average of 62 years. Hirota et al. [13] found that the male to female ratio was about 2:1. The adenomas are located primarily in the antrum. Histologically, the adenomas of the stomach resemble those of the intestines. They are composed of glandular structures lined with tall columnar cells most of which do not secrete mucus and may have a short striated border. The mucus that some cells secrete is in large part acidic sialomucin which is normally present in the small intestine but not the stomach. The mucous cells are usually goblet shaped. Paneth cells and argentaffin cells may also be present. These cells indicate that the adenomas are generally made of cells with intestinal features [28]. They appear to have originated in the metaplastic mucosa as evidenced by the common association of intestinal metaplasia in the surrounding mucosa. These polyps have also been called metaplastic polyps [21] which may, however, be confused with the metaplastic polyp of the colon, an entirely different type of lesion. Rarely, the adenoma may be composed of gastric type cells with the secretion of only the neutral type of glycoprotein. The gastric type adenoma is very rare, 4% of adenomas in Hirota's series [13]. Incidences of different types of adenoma vary. While in Japan the flat adenoma is about three times more common than the papillary adenoma, the reverse seems to be true in the United States.

Flat Adenoma

As the name implies, the flat adenoma does not form a nodular mass. The flat surface is slightly irregular, resembling the contour of a flower bed. In the vast majority of cases, the adenoma is slightly raised above the mucosal surface, resembling the type 2A early carcinoma of the stomach, thus it has also been called 2A-like lesion. Rarely, its surface is even with the surface of the surrounding mucosa (2B-like lesion) or slightly depressed (2C-like lesion) [32]. Irrespective of whether they are slightly elevated or depressed there is a characteristic histological pattern. There is usually a two-tier appearance in that the adenomatous tissue occupies the superficial 50%–70% of the mucosa whereas the deep portion of the lesion is composed of nonneoplastic glandular tissue (Fig. 1). The adenomatous glands are tubular in shape, thus the flat adenoma has been called, in the WHO classification, "tubular adenoma" [35]. The lining cells of the glands are slender, having basally located nuclei which are elongated, uniform and closely packed in a "picket fence" fashion. The majority of the cells are not mucus-secreting. There is very little pleomorphism and mitotic figures are rare. Goblet cells and Paneth cells may be present. The glands underneath the adenomatous tissue are often dilated, even cystic, and show intestinal metaplasia which is commonly of the incomplete type. The flat adenomas usually occur as a single lesion. In a series reported by Watanabe [47] 50 of a total of 75 cases had single adenomas, 19 had two adenomas, 5 had three adenomas, and one had 5 adenomas. Flat adenomas are usually small, 80% of them less than 2 cm in diameter [13].

Compared to the papillary adenoma, the flat adenoma shows a much lower grade of dysplasia and less proliferative activity. It is not surprising, therefore, that the lesion is often stationary. Kamiya et al. [18] followed 85

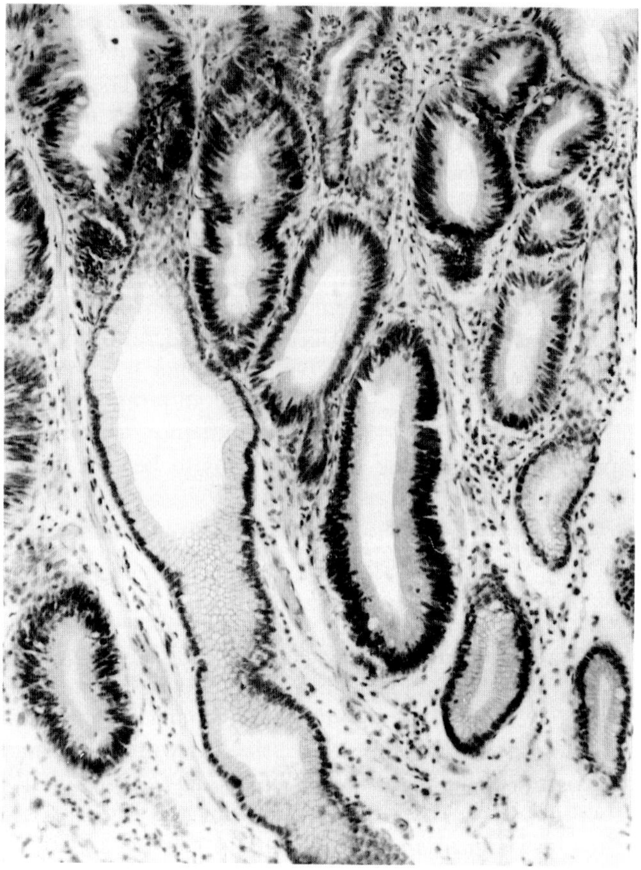

Fig. 1. Flat adenoma. The adenomatous glands are lined by densely packed slender cells. The nuclei are elongated and arranged in a picket-fence fashion. In comparison, the cells in the nonadenomatous glands have short nuclei and abundant cytoplasm. One long gland is dilated. ×120

lesions in 74 patients for 6 months to 12 years. Only eight lesions showed gross changes, four becoming larger and four smaller. None, however, disappeared. Because of the relatively low growth activity this lesion has been called "atypical epithelium" or "borderline lesion" [30, 43]. It must be borne in mind that these terms are commonly applied to benign but uncertain lesions of a heterogeneous nature. They simply mean that the lesion is neither benign nor malignant and thus, as currently used, their meaning is the same as that of dysplasia. The terms can be applied to adenomatous as well as nonneoplastic tissue seen in a variety of benign conditions such as chronic atrophic gastritis and postgastrectomy stump. The dysplastic cells in the latter situations may revert to normal whereas a true adenoma is nonreversible. One important differentiating feature is that an adenoma is a localized, well defined, and grossly visible lesion, whereas the nonneoplastic dysplastic epithelium can only be seen microscopically, occurs in multiple areas, and shows varying degrees of cellular abnormalities.

Papillary Adenoma

Papillary adenomas are large nodular lesions. Their average size is about 4 cm in diameter [27] although adenomas as large as 15 cm in diameter have been reported [38]. They may be sessile or have a short pedicle. Adenomas with a long pedicle, seen in the large intestine, are rare in the stomach. The contour of the adenoma is nodular and lobulated, with deep crevices which can be seen in the radiological examination. Although grossly villous adenoma is uncommon in the stomach, microscopic villous pattern is a frequent component of papillary adenoma in the stomach. Compared to those in the flat adenoma, the cells in the papillary adenoma show much more pleomorphism; the cells are larger, and so are the nuclei (Fig. 2). There is psuedostratification. The nuclei are oval rather than slender, with coarse chromatin pattern. Mitoses are common. The plump appearance of the cells and higher degree of dysplasia make the papillary adenoma of the stomach identical to that seen in the intestines. The cells, like those in the intestinal adenoma, are often not mucus-secreting and those which do secrete mucus are usually goblet-shaped. The mucin is of the acidic type, principally sialomucin, but also sulphomucin. Benign nonneoplastic glands, sometimes dilated, may be present at the base of the adenoma. Most frequently, however, the adenomatous tissue extends through the full thickness of the mucosa to the level of muscularis mucosae. Paneth cells are rare. Also present are occasional cells of an endocrine nature. Gastrin, somatostatin and glicentin secretions have all been reported [14].

The age and sex distribution as well as the location and the number of papillary adenomas do not differ from those of the flat adenoma. Papillary adenomas are, however, clearly more dysplastic than flat adenomas, and have higher proliferative activity. The mucosa surrounding the papillary adenoma also frequently shows intestinal metaplasia. However, metaplastic change is usually of the complete type.

Nonneoplastic Polyp

The nonneoplastic polyps of the stomach are much more frequent than the adenomatous lesions. They are characterized by the nearly normal epithelial cells lining the glandular structure. Some of the polyps may develop superficial erosions at the tip. In such regions the epithelium may show regenerative changes with immature proliferating cells which nevertheless can be easily differentiated from the adenomatous cells described above.

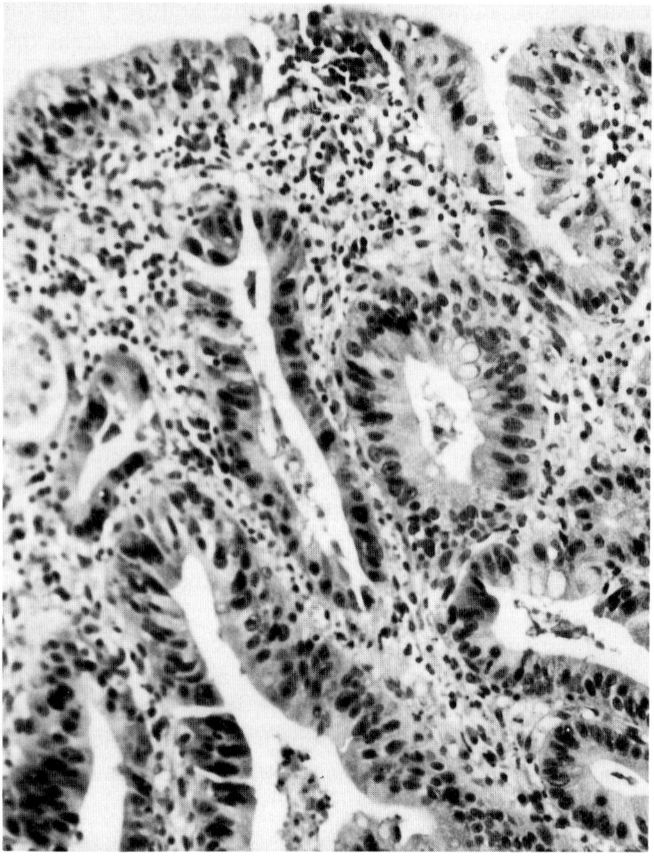

Fig. 2. Papillarey adenoma. The glands are lined by pseudostratified cells which show evident pleomorphism and reduced cytoplasm. The nuclei are plump and oval. A few goblet cells are present. ×200

Hyperplastic Polyp

Hyperplastic polyps are the most common polyps in the stomach, constituting about 75%–90% of all gastric polyps [25]. They are small, usually dome shaped, hemispherical nodules. The surface is mostly smooth but may be superficially eroded, and there is usually no pedicle. They average about 1 cm in diameter, although, rarely, they may be as large as 12 cm [9]. The larger ones may have a papillary appearance similar to that of a papillary adenoma but the hyperplastic polyp has a softer consistency and the lobules have a smooth surface. The polyps are multiple in about 50% of patients. The multiple polyps often appear uniform in size as well as in shape. Their location is random. When they occur in the body of the stomach, polyps typically sit on top of the mucosal folds. In rare cases more than 50 polyps may occur. Such cases have been called hyperplastic polyposis [37].

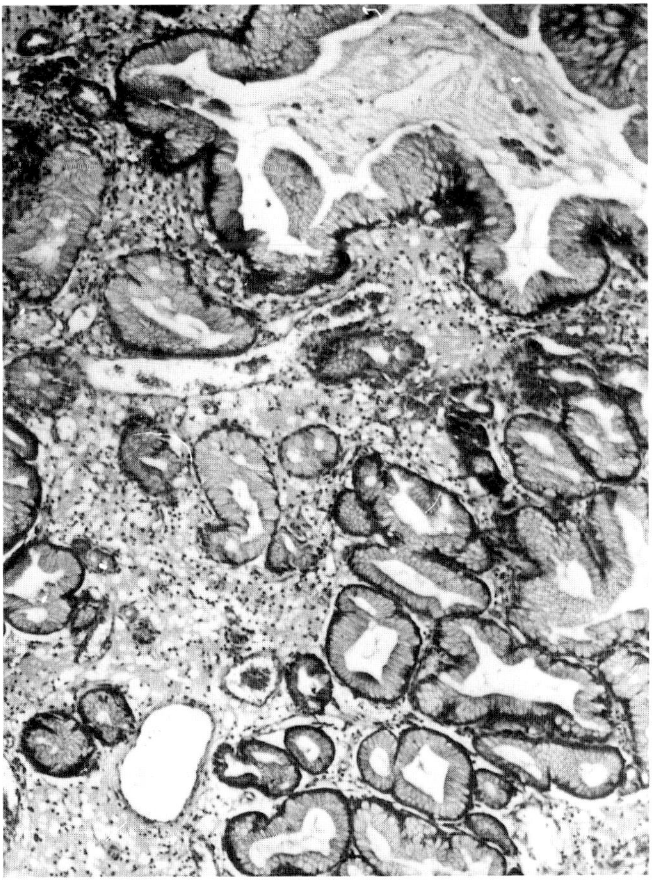

Fig. 3. Hyperplastic polyp. The glands show varying degrees of dilatation. The lining cells appear normal. The edematous stroma is infiltrated by lymphocytes. ×120

Microscopically, the hyperplastic polyps are composed mostly of dilated foveolae and pyloric-type glands (Fig. 3). The smaller and presumably earlier hyperplastic polyps are composed primarily of dilated foveolae only. The descriptive term "polypoid foveolar hyperplasia" has been applied to these lesions [8, 20]. In the well developed hyperplastic polyps, pyloric-type glands are usually present in the deeper portion, even if the polyp occurs in the fundic mucosa. These glands vary in number and are irregular in arrangement. In some polyps a large number of such glands may be closely packed so as to superficially resemble the pattern of an adenoma. The terms "highly differentiated adenoma" [8] and "hyperplastic adenomatous polyp" [20] have sometimes been applied to such cases. In terms of biological potential, these different histological patterns merely represent variants of hyperplastic polyps.

The dilated foveolae are lined by mucus-secreting columnar cells like those seen in the normal stomach. Mitosis is usually absent. There is, however, hyperplasia of such cells so that intraglandular infoldings are common. In the eroded area, the epithelial cells may be immature because of regenerative changes in response to inflammation. Rarely, the mucous cells become excessively enlarged and globoid in shape because of an apparent increase of mucus in the cytoplasm. The mucus in these globoid cells often stains as sialomucin. The nuclei are displaced to the cell membrane and are often irregularly located, giving rise to the appearance of signet-ring cells. Such cellular changes have been called globoid dysplasia, which has been implicated as a possible precursor of signet-ring cell carcinoma [2]. Actual occurrence of signet-ring cell carcinoma in a hyperplastic polyp has not been reported. The significance of the globoid change is therefore uncertain.

The stroma of the hyperplastic polyp is often edematous and loosely fibrous, and contains a varying number of chronic inflammatory cells, mainly small lymphocytes. Occasionally lymphoid nodules may be present but without germinal centers. If the surface area at the dome of the polyp is eroded then there will be infiltration by neutrophils. Within the stroma, strands of smooth muscle cells are often present, usually in small numbers and only at the base of the polyp; in this the hyperplastic polyp differs from the hamartomatous polyp in which the muscle cells often extend to the upper part of the polyp. These muscle cells are connected with the muscularis mucosae, apparently as a result of regenerative proliferation. They form slender bundles which taper off as they grow toward the upper portion of the polyp.

Intestinal metaplasia occurs only infrequently in the upper portion of the hyperplastic polyp. The surrounding mucosa of the polyp shows nonspecific chronic inflammation similar to that seen in the polyp itself. Metaplastic changes also are usually absent. While the neoplastic cells in the adenoma end abruptly as they meet the nonneoplastic neighboring cells, there is no demarcating line between the hyperplastic polyp and the adjacent mucosa.

Hamartomatous Polyp

The hamartomatous polyp is defined as a polyp composed of tissues which are normally present at the location. Although the cells are cytologically normal, the arrangement is usually disorganized. It can be further classified according to its component tissue.

Peutz-Jeghers Polyp

Peutz-Jeghers polyp is a prototype of hamartomatous polyps in the gastrointestinal tract. It occurs in patients with Peutz-Jeghers syndrome

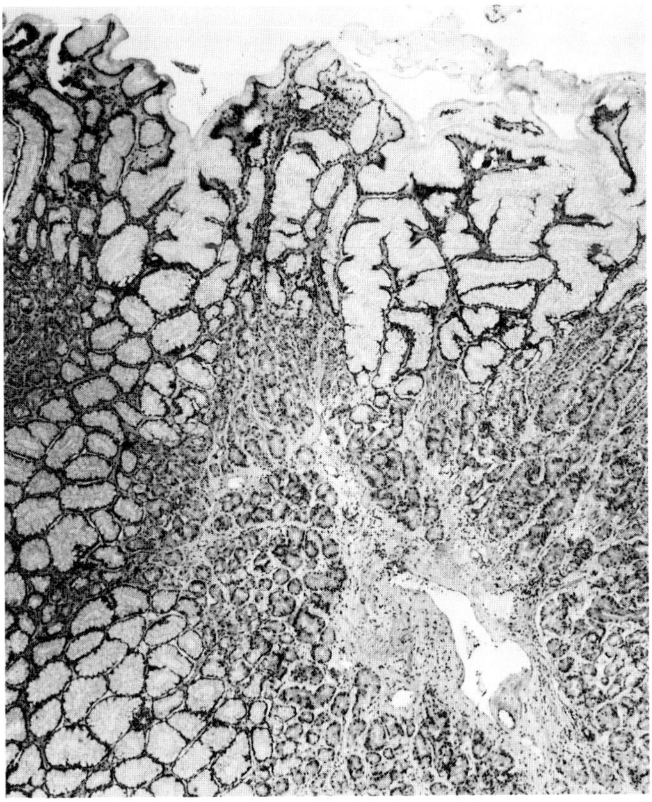

Fig. 4. Peutz-Jeghers polyp. The glands show dilated foveolae, but are otherwise essentially normal. There is no inflammation. ×50

which characteristically has two components: (a) the presence of polyps in the gastrointestinal tract, and (b) melanin pigmentation of the skin and the mucous membrane, most prominently involving the face and the oral cavity. Peutz-Jeghers syndrome is a familial disease with dominant inheritance pattern. The polyps may occur anywhere along the gastrointestinal tract, most frequently in the small intestine. In the stomach they are usually small, multiple and asymptomatic. They are composed of normal mucosal tissue, fundic glands in the fundic mucosa and pyloric glands in the antral mucosa (Fig. 4). The glands are often elongated and may be slightly dilated. There is, however, no intraglandular infolding of the epithelium. The stroma characteristically contains bundles of smooth muscle fibers with varying thickness. These bundles extend from the muscularis mucosae to the surface of the polyp and are not associated with any inflammatory change in the stroma. The epithelial cells in the polyp appear entirely normal, showing no dysplastic or actively proliferative changes. Peutz-Jeghers syndrome is usually diagnosed at an early age, in the second or third decade of life. The syndrome may not be complete in that occasional members of the family may have only the polyps or the pigmentation. Occasionally this type of polyp is seen in non-familial cases.

Juvenile Polyp

The juvenile polyp most commonly occurs as isolated polyp in the colon or rectum in children. These polyps are smooth-surfaced and small and are histologically characterized by the presence of dilated glandular cysts and edematous loose fibrous stroma with many lymphocytes. Because of the retention of mucus in the dilated glands, these polyps are also known as retention polyps. These cases are not hereditary, and the polyps are possibly the result of inflammation. Morson (1962), noting the resemblance of the stromal tissue in the polyp to that of the normal juvenile colon, considered the juvenile polyps to be hamartomas. This possibility is enhanced in the hereditary cases which are manifested sometimes in infants. In these hereditary cases there are many such polyps, which may be limited to the colon or may be present also in the stomach and in the small intestine. The former condition with polyps in the colon only is known as juvenile polyposis coli and the latter as juvenile gastrointestinal polyposis. In the stomach the polyps have dilated glands that are composed primarily of foveolae; but the deep glands are usually reduced in number. The stroma is loosely fibrous and contains lymphocytes. Thus the juvenile polyps of the stomach resemble hyperplastic polyps.

Fundic Gland Polyp

As the name implies these polyps occur in the fundic mucosa of the stomach. They are characterized by the presence of fundic gland proper with parietal cells and chief cells. Most of the glands appear normal or only slightly dilated. Some glands, however, may show marked dilatation, and so such polyps have also been known as glandular cysts [6]. The cytologically normal appearance of the cells identifies these polyps as hamartomatous. However, it has been observed that sometimes the polyps disappear, and some investigators consider them not hamartomatous but merely the result of physiological and functional glandular dilatation [6]. Fundic gland polyps have been associated with familial polyposis coli and Gardner's syndrome [45, 48]. However, cases without polyposis syndrome have been reported in recent years [6, 38a].

Inflammatory Polyp

Inflammatory polyps show prominent chronic inflammation or granulation tissue formation, with or without glandular changes. This type of polyp may be called pseudopolyp. A special form of inflammatory polyp is the inflammatory fibroid polyp which is made entirely of fibrous tissue containing varying amounts of inflammatory cells. Another form of inflammatory polyp is seen in patients with Cronkhite-Canada syndrome [19]. In this nonhereditary syndrome, which occurs primarily in elderly patients, the polyps have dilated glands. There are many polyps throughout the gastrointestinal tract and the major symptom is diarrhea.

Heterotopic Polyp

Heterotopic polyps are made of normal-appearing glands seen in the neighboring organs such as Brunner glands of the duodenum and the pancreatic parenchyma. Brunner gland polyps occur primarily in the pyloric region and, if big, cause obstruction [17]. The heterotopic pancreatic tissue is primarily a submucosal lesion that may become distinctly polypoid and ulcerated, and bleed as a result [50]. Heterotopic pancreatic tissue may have exocrine as well as endocrine tissues.

Relation of Gastric Polyp to Gastric Carcinoma

Gastric polyps have been known to be closely related to gastric carcinoma for many years. The first detailed description of the association was made by Ménétrier in 1888 [23]. He recognized two types of gross morphology. In one there are multiple discrete polyps in the stomach, to which he gave the name polyadenomes polypeux (polypoid adenomas). His illustrations indicate that these so-called adenomas were hyperplastic polyps. The second type is shown as a diffuse thickening of the gastric mucosa resembling the appearance of ruffled cloth, and this type he called polyadenomes en nappe (cloth-like adenomas), now known as Ménétrier's disease. Ménétrier [23] described an ulcerated gastric carcinoma accompanied by multiple "polypoid adenomas". It is not clear, however, whether the carcinoma had originated from the polyp or merely accompanied the polyp in the intervening mucosa. Uncertainty regarding the origin of the carcinoma in the presence of gastric polyps dominated the old literature, resulting in a wide variation in the reported incidence of carcinoma in patients with gastric polyps. This varied from 0% to as high as 51% [21a]. The polyp was variously called adenoma or polyp, without histological clarification. It was in 1965 that Ming and Goldman [27] made the first attempt to classify the gastric polyps by their histological and cytological characteristics, and thus they described two basic forms of gastric polyp. One was named regenerative polyp and was characterized by dilated foveolae with normal-appearing epithelial cells and inflammatory stroma. This type of polyp is now known as hyperplastic polyp. The second form of gastric polyp resembles the adenoma of the colon with dysplastic cells but no inflammatory changes. This type of polyp is truly adenomatous. They also pointed out that malignant change within the polyp itself occurs frequently in the adenoma but not in the regenerative polyp. However, malignant change may occur in the intervening gastric mucosa outside both of these polyps.

Malignant Change in Polyp

Adenoma

In view of the dysplastic nature of the cells in adenoma, it is to be expected that malignant change in gastric adenomas will be common. It has been pointed out (see "Flat Adenoma", p. 33) that flat adenomas are composed of cells with low grade dysplasia and low proliferative activity whereas the papillary adenoma has a high grade of dysplasia and active proliferation. The incidence of malignant change within them is consistent with these cellular characteristics. The reported incidences of malignant change in the papillary adenomas varied from 13% [9] to 76% [31] and those in the flat adenomas were between 5% [32] and 14% [13]. The average incidence of malignant change within the adenomas is 34% when calculated by the number of adenomas and 25% by the number of cases (Table 2).

Hyperplastic Polyp

Since the recognition of hyperplastic polyp as a distinct entity, it has been generally agreed that this type of polyp has no malignant potential. This view is understandable since the polyp is composed of cells which appear normal. However, there have been sporadic reports of malignant change in the hyperplastic polyp. The average reported frequency of malignant change in hyperplastic polyps remains low: 1.0% of polyps and 1.7% of cases

Table 2. Average frequency of malignant change in gastric polyps, and average frequency of coexisting gastric carcinoma

	Frequency of malignant change				Frequency of coexisting carcinoma			
	Polyps		Cases		Polyps		Cases	
	%	Number	%	Number	%	Number	%	Number
Adenoma	34	272/808	25	25/101	48	52/108	49	141/288
Hyperplastic polyp	1.0	34/3526	1.7	11/660			13	70/533

Source of data: Daibo et al. [5], Ghazi et al. [9], Hattori [12], Hirota et al. [13], Kozuka et al. [21], Laxen et al. [22], Ming [25], Nagayo [31], Nakamura [33], Nakamura and Nakano [34], Nakamura et al. [32], Snover [40], Yamagata and Hisamichi [49]

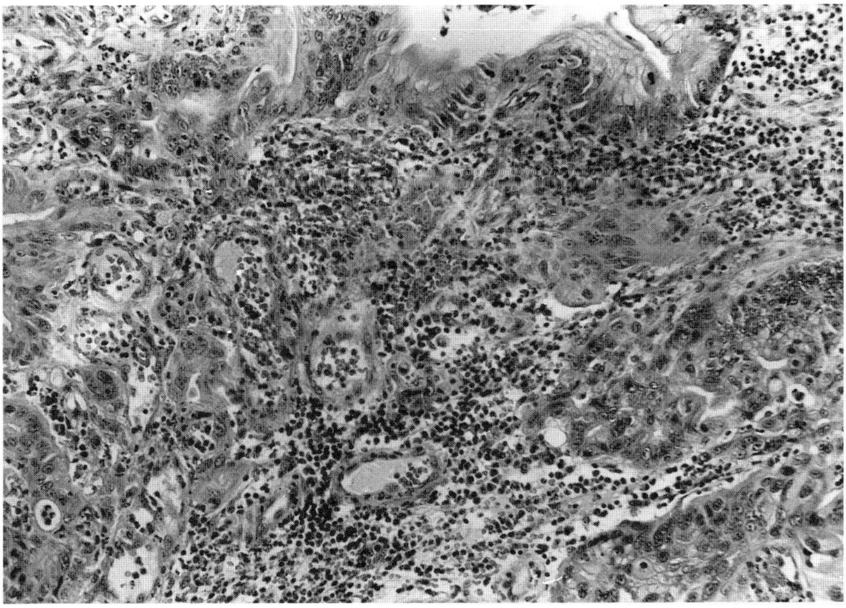

Fig. 5. Carcinoma in a hyperplastic polyp. This small focus of adenocarcinoma was found in a superficial region of the polyp where dysplasia was present in the adjoining glands. ×150

(Table 2). Even these low percentages were at first difficult to explain in view of the totally innocuous appearance of the cells in such polyps. Personal review of the histology of such cases has left the author in no doubt, however, that carcinoma does occur in the hyperplastic polyp (Fig. 5), although only rarely [26]. It is also evident that the carcinomatous change occurs in a dysplastic or adenomatous area which may be located at the tip of the polyp, but may also be randomly located. Evidently the malignant change in a hyperplastic polyp goes through a stage of dysplasia or adenomatous alteration first. Similar experience has been reported by others in recent years [5, 12, 20]. So far there have been no reports of instances in which the carcinoma in a hyperplastic polyp has metastasized or invaded the submucosal tissue. It can still be stated, therefore, that, in practice, hyperplastic polyps are generally innocuous and have a low possibility of malignant change. However, it is clear that thorough histological examination of the polyp is important, not only to differentiate it from the adenoma but also to identify the presence of dysplastic or carcinomatous tissue within it. Excisional biopsy of these polyps is therefore necessary.

Hamartomatous Polyp

Malignant change in the hamartomatous polyp is about as unlikely as in the hyperplastic polyp. There have been sporadic reports of gastrointestinal malignancy in patients with Peutz-Jeghers syndrome [11, 46]. The characteristically normal-appearing tissue in such polyps again makes it difficult to explain the malignant change. In most reports it is not clear whether the carcinoma had indeed occurred within the polyp or resided outside the polyp. In most cases, at the time of diagnosis, the carcinoma was large whereas the coexisting Peutz-Jeghers polyps were small. It is known that polyps of the colon in Peutz-Jeghers syndrome may be adenomatous, and carcinoma may develop in such an adenoma. Although no adenoma has been reported in the stomach of patients with this syndrome, dysplastic lesion in a gastric polyp with carcinoma has been reported [3]. In any case, there is an increased incidence of carcinoma in the gastrointestinal tract of the Peutz-Jeghers syndrome patients. Furthermore, the age of these patients with carcinoma is much younger than that of similar patients in the general population. The average age of patients with gastric carcinoma in the former group was only 27 years [12].

The question of malignancy in juvenile polyposis patients is even less clear. It is known that, rarely, carcinoma may develop in such patients as well as members of their family who do not have polyps [41]. In most cases the carcinoma was found in adenomatous or dysplastic lesions in the colon, only rarely in the stomach [1, 10, 10a]. I have personally seen a case of carcinoma in an area of dysplasia in a gastric juvenile polyp (Fig. 6) in a patient who had multiple juvenile polyps in the stomach as well as the intestinal tract.

The fundic gland polyp is also composed of normal-appearing glands. As mentioned above, fundic gland polyps occur in association with familial polyposis coli and Gardner's syndrome. It is known that, in such cases, adenoma and carcinoma may develop in the stomach as well as the small intestine [4, 16]. Carcinoma in the stomach, however, has not been related to the fundic gland polyp; neither have there been reports of dysplastic changes in such polyps.

Inflammatory and Heterotopic Polyps

Carcinoma does not occur in inflammatory polyps [22]. Rare carcinomas occurring in the ectopic pancreas have been reported [12a].

Coexisting Gastric Carcinoma

Stomachs containing polyps may have independent coexisting carcinomas. In the case of adenomas, the reported incidence of such carcinomas varies from 3.4% to 70%. The lowest incidence occurred in 1 of 29 cases [22] and

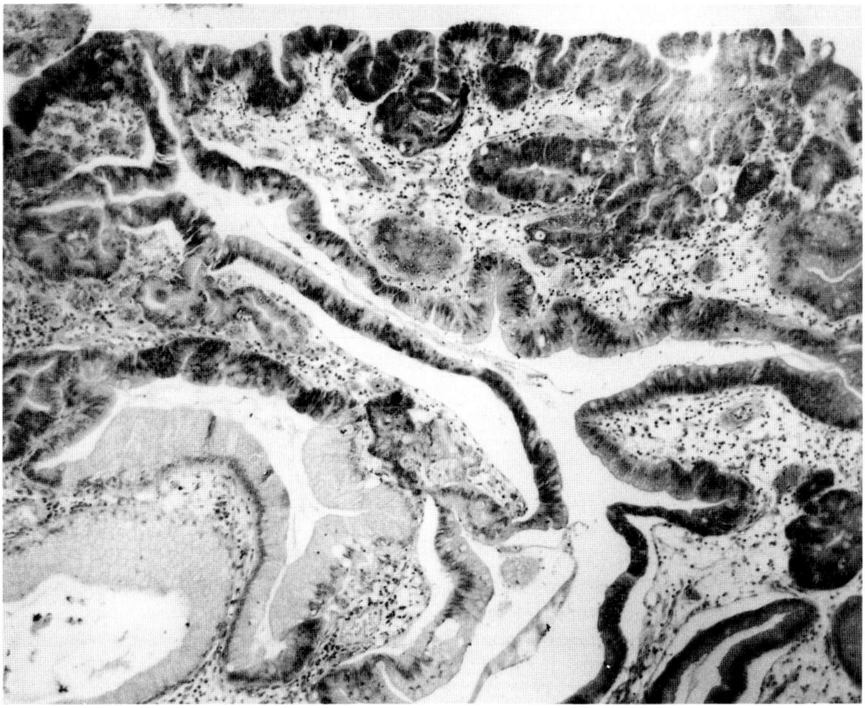

Fig. 6. Carcinoma in a juvenile polyp. A focus of adenocarcinoma is shown at the upper center. The dilated glands underneath are dysplastic. ×150

the highest in 84 of 121 cases [13]. The average incidence is about 49% (Table 2).

Coexisting carcinoma occurred in 4.5% to 28% of cases of hyperplastic polyp. The lowest incidence reported was 9 of 198 cases [22] and the highest 21 of 74 cases [44]. The average is 13% (Table 2). In hamartomatous polyposis cases, as discussed above with regard to malignant change within the polyp, the incidence of coexisting carcinoma cannot be evaluated. It is clear, however, that gastrointestinal carcinomas occur with increased frequency in the patients with familial polyposis syndrome. In 130 cases with inflammatory polyps reported by Laxen et al. [22], gastric carcinoma outside the polyp was found in three cases.

Summary

It is evident that gastric adenoma is a distinctly premalignant lesion. The adenoma must be excised and carefully examined for possible malignant change. The incidence of malignant change in hyperplastic and hamartomatous polyps is low. Nevertheless, there is a distinct possibility of such occurrences, particularly if dysplastic or adenomatous tissue is present within the polyp. It is therefore also necessary to examine these polyps histologically. It is important, too, to consider the possibility of coexisting, but independent, carcinoma in stomachs containing polyps. Nearly 50% of patients with gastric adenoma have independent carcinomas of the stomach. About 13% of those with hyperplastic polyps have separate carcinoma in the stomach. This incidence is significant. It is therefore important that whenever there is a polyp in the stomach, the entire gastric mucosa must be examined to rule out a coexisting carcinoma. When this is done, the chance of finding an early gastric carcinoma is high. In the report by Hirota et al. [13], 84 of 121 cases of gastric adenoma had coexisting carcinoma, 55 early and 29 advanced.

References

1. Beacham DH, Shields HM, Raffensperger EC, Enterline HT (1978) Juvenile and adenomatous gastrointestinal polyposis. Am J Dig Dis 23:1137–1143
2. Borchard F (1986) Precancerous conditions and lesions of the stomach. In: Rugge M, Arslan-Pagnini C, DiMario F (eds) Carcinoma gastrico e lesioni precancerose dello stomaco. Unicopi Milan, pp 175–210
3. Cochet B, Carrol J, Desbeillets L, Widgren S (1979) Peutz-Jeghers syndrome associated with gastrointestinal carcinoma. Gut 20:169–175
4. Coffey RJ Jr, Knight CD Jr, van Heerden JA, Weiland LH (1985) Gastric adenocarcinoma complicating Gardner's syndrome in a North American Woman. Gastroenterology 88(1):1263–1266
5. Daibo M, Itabashi M, Hirota T (1987) Malignant transformation of gastric hyperplastic polyps. Am J Gastroenterol 82:1016–1025
6. Eidt S, Stolte M (1989) Gastric glandular cysts – investigations into their genesis and relationship to colorectal epithelial tumors. Z Gastroenterol 27:212–217
7. Elsborg L, Andersen D, Myhere-Jensen O, Bastrup-Madsen P (1977) Gastric mucosal polyps in pernicious anaemia. Scand J Gastroenterol 12:49–52
8. Elster K (1976) Histologic classification of gastric polyps. Curr Top Pathol 65:77–93
9. Ghazi A, Ferstenberg H, Shinya H (1984) Endoscopic gastroduodenal polypectomy. Ann Surg 200:175–180
10. Goodman ZD, Yardley JH, Milligan FD (1979) Pathogenesis of colonic polyps in multiple juvenile polyposis: report of a case associated with gastric polyps and carcinoma of the rectum. Cancer 43:1906–1913

10a. Grigioni WF, Alampi G, Martinelli G, Piccoluga A (1981) Atypical juvenile polyposis. Histopathology 5:361–376

11. Halbert RE (1982) Peutz-Jeghers syndrome with metastasizing gastric adenocarcinoma. Report of a case. Arch Pathol Lab Med 106:517–520
12. Hattori T (1985) Morphological range of hyperplastic polyps and carcinomas arising in hyperplastic polyps of the stomach. J Clin Pathol 38:622–630

12a. Hickman DM, Frey CF, Carson JW (1981) Adenocarcinoma arising in gastric heterotopic pancreas. West J Med 135:57–62

13. Hirota T, Okada T, Itabashi M, Kitaoka H (1984) Histogenesis of human gastric cancer – with special reference to the significance of adenoma as a precancerous lesion. In: Ming SC (ed) Precursors of gastric cancer. Praeger, Philadelphia, pp 233–252

14. Ito H, Yokozaki H, Hata J, Mandai K, Tahara E (1984) Glicentin-containing cells in intestinal metaplasia, adenoma and carcinoma of the stomach. Virchows Arch [A] 404:17–29
15. Janunger K, Domellof L (1978) Gastric polyps and precancerous mucosal changes after partial gastrectomy. Acta Chir Scand 144:293–298
16. Jarvinen H, Nyberg M, Peltokallio P (1983) Upper gastrointestinal tract polyps in familial adenomatosis. Gut 24:333–339
17. Johnson CD, Bynum TE (1976) Brunner gland heterotopia presenting as gastric antral polyps. Gastrointest Endosc 22:210–211
18. Kamiya T, Morishita T, Asakura H, Miura S, Munakata Y, Tsuchiya M (1982) Long term follow-up on gastric adenoma and its relation to gastric protruded carcinoma. Cancer 50:2493–2503
19. Kindblom LG, Angervall L, Santesson B, Selander S (1977) Cronkhite-Canada syndrome. Case report. Cancer 39:2651–2657
20. Koch HK, Lesch R, Cremer M, Oehlert W (1979) Polyp and polypoid foveolar hyperplasia in gastric biopsy specimens and their precancerous prevalence. Front Gastrointest Res 4:183–191
21. Kozuka S, Masamoto K, Suzuki S, Kubota K, Yokoyama Y (1977) Histogenetic types and size of polypoid lesion of the stomach, with special reference to cancerous changes. Gan 68:267–274
21a. Lawrence JC (1936) Gastrointestinal polyps: statistical study of malignancy incidence. Am J Surg 31:499–505
22. Laxen F, Sipponen P, Ihamaki T, Hakkiluoto A, Dortscheva Z (1982) Gastric polyps; their morphological and endoscopical characteristics and relation to gastric carcinoma. Acta Pathol Microbiol Scand [A] 90:221–228
23. Ménétrier P (1888) Des polyadénomes gastriques et de leurs rapport avec le cancer de l'estomac. Arch Physiol Norm Pathol 1:32–55, 236–262
24. Ming SC (1973) Tumors of the esophagus and stomach. Armed Forces Institute of Pathology, Washington, pp 99–101 (Atlas of tumor pathology, 2nd Ser, fasc 7)
25. Ming SC (1977) The classification and significance of gastric polyps. In: Yardley JH, Morson BM (eds) The gastrointestinal tract. Williams and Wilkins, Baltimore, pp 149–175
26. Ming SC (1984) Malignant potential of epithelial polyps of the stomach. In: Ming SC (ed) Precursors of gastric cancer. Praeger, Philadelphia, pp 219–231
27. Ming SC, Goldman H (1965) Gastric polyps: a histogenetic classification and its relation to carcinoma. Cancer 18:721–726
28. Morson BC (1955) Gastric polyps composed of intestinal epithelium. Br J Cancer 9:550–557
29. Morson BC (1962) Some peculiarities in the histology of intestinal polyps. Dis Colon Rectum 5:337–344
30. Nagayo T (1971) Histological diagnosis of biopsied gastric mucosa with special reference to that of borderline lesions. Gann Monogr Cancer Res 11:245–256
31. Nagayo T (1986) Histogenesis and precursors of human gastric cancer. Springer, Berlin Heidelberg New York, pp 103–111
32. Nakamura K, Sagakuchi H, Enjoji M (1988) Depressed adenoma of the stomach. Cancer 62:2197–2202
33. Nakamura T (1970) Pathohistologische Einteilung der Magenpolypen mit spezifischer Betrachtung ihrer malignen Entartung. Chirurg 41:122–130
34. Nakamura T, Nakano G (1985) Histopathological classification and malignant change in gastric polyps. J Clin Pathol 38:754–764
35. Oota K, Sobin LH (1977) Histological typing of gastric and oesophageal tumours. World Health Organization, Geneva, p 37 (International histological classification of tumours, no 18)
36. Ovaska JT, Ekfors TO, Havia TV, Kujari HP (1986) Endoscopic follow-up after resection for gastric or duodenal ulcer. Acta Chir Scand 152:289–295
37. Rosch W (1980) Epidemiology, pathogenesis, diagnosis, treatment of benign gastric tumours. Front Gastrointest Res 6:167–184

38. Shauffer IA, O'Conner SJ (1966) Villous tumor of the stomach. Radiology 86: 734–735
38a. Sipponen P, Laxen F, Seppala K (1983) Cystic "hamartomatous" gastric polyps: a disorder of oxyntic glands. Histopathology 7:729–737
39. Siurala M (1981) Gastritis, its fate and sequelae. Ann Clin Res 13:111–113
40. Snover DC (1985) Benign epithelial polyps of the stomach. Pathol Annu 20(1): 303–329
41. Stemper TJ, Kent TH, Summers RW (1975) Juvenile polyposis and gastrointestinal carcinoma. A study of a kindred. Ann Intern Med 83:639–646
42. Stockbrugger RW, Menon GG, Beilby JO, Mason RR, Cotton PB (1983) Gastroscopic screening in 80 patients with pernicious anaemia. Gut 24:1141–1147
43. Sugano H, Nakamura K, Takagi K (1971) An atypical epithelium of the stomach. A clinicopathological entity. Gann Monogr Cancer Res 11:257–269
44. Tomasulo J (1971) Gastric polyps; histologic types and their relationship to gastric carcinoma. Cancer 27:1346–1355
45. Tonelli F, Nardi F, Bechi P, Taddei G, Gozzo P, Romagnoli P (1985) Extracolonic polyps in familial polyposis coli and Gardner's syndrome. Dis Colon Rectum 28: 664–668
46. Utsunomiya J, Gocho H, Miyanaga T, Hamaguchi E, Kashimure A, Aoki N, Komatsu I (1975) Peutz-Jeghers syndrome. Its natural course and management. Johns Hopkins Med J 136:71–82
47. Watanabe H (1972) Argentaffin cells in adenoma of the stomach. Cancer 30: 1267–1274
48. Watanabe H, Enjoji M, Yao T, Ohsato K (1978) Gastric lesions in familial adenomatosis coli. Their incidence and histological analysis. Hum Pathol 9:269–283
49. Yamagata S, Hisamichi S (1979) Precancerous lesions of the stomach. World J Surg 3:671–673
50. Yamagiwa H, Ishihara A, Sekoguchi T, Matsuzaki O (1977) Heterotopic pancreas in surgically resected stomach. Gastroenterol Jpn 12:380–386

5 Is Intestinal Metaplasia of Gastric Mucosa a Precancerous Lesion?

J. R. Jass

Historical Perspectives

Following the first description of intestinalized epithelium within gastric mucosa [34], there was disagreement as to whether this lesion represented a congenital or an acquired heterotopia. Schmidt [73] noted the association of gastritis and intestinalized mucosa, but others regarded intestinal foci as congenital ectopias [2, 89]. The last interpretation was based on the observation of intestinal type foci within seemingly normal gastric mucosa. Moreover, such foci showed an extremely close resemblance to normal small intestinal mucosa. Indeed, electron microscopic studies have shown that normal small intestine and intestinalized foci within gastric mucosa may be indistinguishable [69].

Others argued that intestinalization represented an acquired lesion, arising through faulty regeneration in chronically inflamed gastric mucosa [12, 42]. Magnus [42] was unable to demonstrate foci of intestinalized mucosa with an entirely normal gastric mucosa or in fetal stomach. Subsequently it was shown that the extent of intestinalization increased with age [49, 80, 87].

Following the pioneering work of Cheng and Leblond [4] it is now accepted that all gastrointestinal cell types are derived from a single stem cell. Such cells have been characterized at the electron microscopic level in man, occupying the crypt base or neck region of the gastric glands [70]. It has been suggested that intestinalization arises through aberrant differentiation of this multipotential, stem cell population [45, 83].

It is now accepted that most, if not all, examples of intestinalization within gastric mucosa represent an acquired heterotopia or metaplasia. Furthermore, intestinal metaplasia (IM) is regarded as the final stage of a dynamic inflammatory process – chronic gastritis [12, 92]. The concept of a disease continuum was refined by the introduction of the terms "chronic superficial gastritis", "atrophic gastritis", and "gastric atrophy" [30, 35, 49, 96]. Whitehead et al. [95] further clarified and expanded this purely

Department of Pathology, University of Auckland School of Medicine, Private Bag, Auckland, New Zealand

Ying-Chan Zhang/Keiichi Kawai (Eds.)
Precancerous Conditions and Lesions of the Stomach

morphological classification. More recently, attempts have been made to classify chronic gastritis according to the underlying etiology or pathogenesis [5, 97].

Developmental Biology and Morphogenesis of IM

Metaplasia is defined as the replacement of one tissue by another during postnatal life. IM represents the conversion of gastric type mucosa to mucosa that may closely resemble or be indistinguishable from small intestinal epithelium. Although histopathologists take this lesion for granted, developmental biologists would regard metaplasia as no less remarkable than the inappropriate replacement of a lost arthropod limb by an antenna (a homeotic transformation) [82]. As stated above, IM must be due to an alteration at the level of the stem cell. This will occur during a phase of active tissue growth, for example during regeneration following gastritic injury. However, it is not yet established whether the change in developmental commitment of the stem cell population is due to a somatic mutation or an epigenetic modulation. In either case the change must be heritable on cell division. An interesting nonmutational theory involving biochemical switches has been proposed recently [82]. This theory would be consistent with the view that IM is a form of tissue adaptation reflecting changes in the gastric microenvironment.

IM usually occurs in small islands separated by gastric mucosa showing varying degrees of chronic gastritis. There is evidence that the initial stimulus required for the development of IM often takes the form either of an ulcer or an erosion [50, 63]. Thus metaplastic change would take place within the actively regenerating epithelium relining focal erosions. Repeated cycles of erosion and faulty regeneration would increase the number of metaplastic islands until confluence was achieved. This insight into the pathogenesis of intestinal metaplasia was provided by a detailed microreconstruction study [50]. It helps to explain why IM may sometimes be bordered by near-normal-appearing gastric mucosa.

IM and Gastric Carcinoma

The role of IM in the histogenesis of gastric carcinoma has been debated since the latter part of the nineteenth century. Schmidt [73] noted an association between gastric carcinoma and gastritis. Konjetzny [33] put forward the view that carcinoma never develops in healthy gastric mucosa. Others have regarded IM as precancerous, noting extensive IM in the vicinity of gastric cancers and the presence of intestinal features within tumors themselves [25, 51, 92].

In contrast, Guiss and Stewart [19], Stout [87] and Fairly et al. [13] were unconvinced that IM had any cancerous potential. Stout [87] accepted that IM occurred as an extensive change around carcinomas, but believed this reflected the occurrence of gastric carcinoma in an aged population. He was unable to demonstrate any convincing gradation from benign IM to carcinoma. Fairley et al. [13] followed up patients with chronic gastritis for 5 years and did not detect any increased incidence of gastric carcinoma.

Two papers by Morson [46, 47] marked a turning point in the debate. He showed that age alone did not account for the increased extent of IM in patients with gastric carcinoma [46]. He also illustrated the origin of gastric carcinomas within IM [47]. More recent detailed studies have confirmed the latter finding [29, 59, 72]. Numerous studies have demonstrated intestinal type features within gastric carcinomas. These have utilized light microscopy [25, 51], enzyme histochemistry [32, 64, 93], mucin histochemistry [15, 45] and electron microscopy [25, 60, 71]. In other studies, generally more recent ones, various intestinal tumor markers have been demonstrated in gastric neoplasms. These include carcinoembryonic antigen [3, 11, 76], goblet cell antigen [66] and large intestinal mucin antigen [41].

Long-term prospective studies of patients with chronic gastritis overturned the conclusions of Fairley et al. [13] by showing an increased incidence of gastric carcinoma as compared with control populations [53, 78, 79, 91].

A view gradually emerged that carcinomas arising in IM might represent a distinct histogenetic entity [25, 47, 51]. This idea culminated in a paper by Laurén [36] in which the intestinal-type carcinoma was envisaged to arise in IM and the diffuse type in normal gastric mucosae. He assessed several criteria in his tumor classification including architecture, cytology, mode and type of mucus secretion, pattern of growth, and host tissue response.

The detailed histogenetic studies on examples of early gastric carcinoma by Nakamura et al. [59] supported Laurén's [36] hypothesis. However, the notion that all intestinal-type carcinomas arose in IM and all diffuse carcinomas within normal gastric mucosae was held by many to be an oversimplification [20, 29, 32, 62].

Epidemiological studies have also implicated IM in the histogenesis of gastric carcinoma. IM was shown to be more common in populations at high risk of gastric carcinoma than in age-matched controls from low-risk areas [24]. Furthermore, intestinal-type carcinomas were noted to predominate in high-risk areas [6, 52, 54]. Migration from high- to low-risk areas resulted in a falling incidence of intestinal- but not diffuse-type carcinomas [7]. The latter study was based on Hawaiians of Japanese origin. These findings would appear to support the concept of an environmentally induced IM-carcinoma sequence [5].

In spite of the preceding evidence linking IM and gastric carcinoma, some workers have doubted whether IM should be accepted wholeheartedly as a precancerous lesion [20, 32, 45, 48, 83, 93]. Several studies, in which the distribution of IM was mapped in some detail, have failed to demonstrate a convincing relationship between gastric cancer and IM [67, 84]. Others argued that the presence of metaplastic features within a gastric neoplasm did not necessarily prove that the tumor had originated in IM [32, 45, 83, 93]. Instead, it was suggested that IM might arise within carcinomatous epithelium in a manner analogous to benign intestinalization. In support of this assertion, histochemical and ultrastructural studies have demonstrated intestinal characteristics in virtually all gastric cancers, whether intestinal or diffuse in type [32, 60, 71]. It has also been noted that tissue in IM is highly specialized epithelium and closely resembles the mucosa of the normal small intestine – a membrane in which the development of adenocarcinoma is rare [32]. Finally, and perhaps most importantly, IM is a common lesion, particularly in elderly subjects [46, 81]. Thus, although IM is the most selective marker of malignancy within the entity of chronic gastritis, its high prevalence precludes its practical use as a marker of precancer [48]. Recently gastric dysplasia has been advocated as a more selective marker of increased malignant risk [8, 44, 48, 57, 61].

Heterogeneity of IM

The role of IM as a precancerous lesion has been reevaluated following the demonstration of its different types. As stated above, IM may be indistinguishable from normal small bowel mucosa in terms of its detailed structure and function. However, the appearance of goblet cells in gastric mucosa is not always accompanied by other types of small intestinal cells. Paneth cells may be absent and columnar cells showing varied patterns of differentiation and hybrid features may be seen in the place of mature enterocytes. Such findings have been reported in light microscopic preparations [23, 45, 58] as well as at the ultrastructural level [17, 23, 60, 85, 88]. Mucin histochemical studies have also demonstrated heterogeneity. The goblet cells of IM secrete sialomucins as does the normal small intestine. However, sulfomucin production is well described [15, 18, 38, 39, 83]. Lev [38] noted the secretion of sulfomucin in "atypical" epithelium bordering gastric carcinoma. His illustrations showed an epithelium lined by mucous cells of varying size and morphology. However, he did not connect this observation with IM. Stemmermann [83] reported sulfomucin secretion within columnar cells adjacent to goblet cells.

Sialomucins may be classified into N- or O-acetylated types [9]. The goblet cells of IM secrete mainly N-acetylated sialomucins, like normal duodenal mucosa. Teglbjaerg and Nielsen [90] showed that some variants of IM secrete O-acetylated sialomucins, normally found in the distal small bowel and colon.

Heterogeneity has also been described in relation to the expression of brush border enzymes. In completely differentiated IM, the presence of dis-

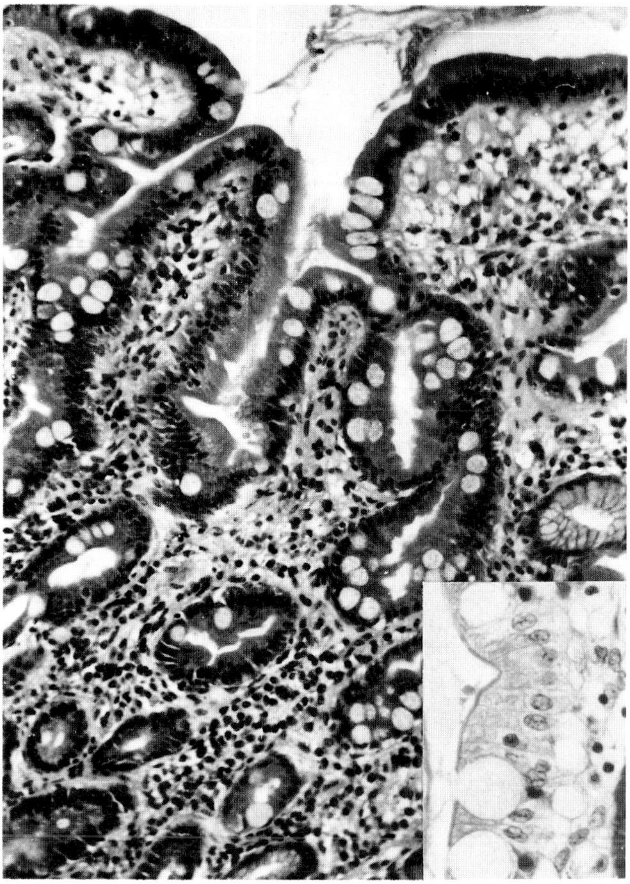

Fig. 1. Complete intestinal metaplasia (IM). The epithelium comprises goblet cells and eosinophilic enterocytes. *Inset* (×300) shows refractile brush border of enterocytes. H & E, ×100

accharidases, alkaline phosphatase, trehalase, and leucine aminopeptidase may be demonstrated [16]. However, enzyme activities may be reduced or absent in incompletely differentiated forms of IM [1, 21, 31, 58, 86].

Classification of IM

The above-mentioned observations regarding the complex heterogeneity of IM were unified by a simple classification of IM into two major types: complete (type I) and incomplete (type II) [26]. Type I IM shows the full complement of intestinal characteristics, closely resembling normal small intestine (or less frequently colon) (Figs. 1, 2). In type II IM the typical

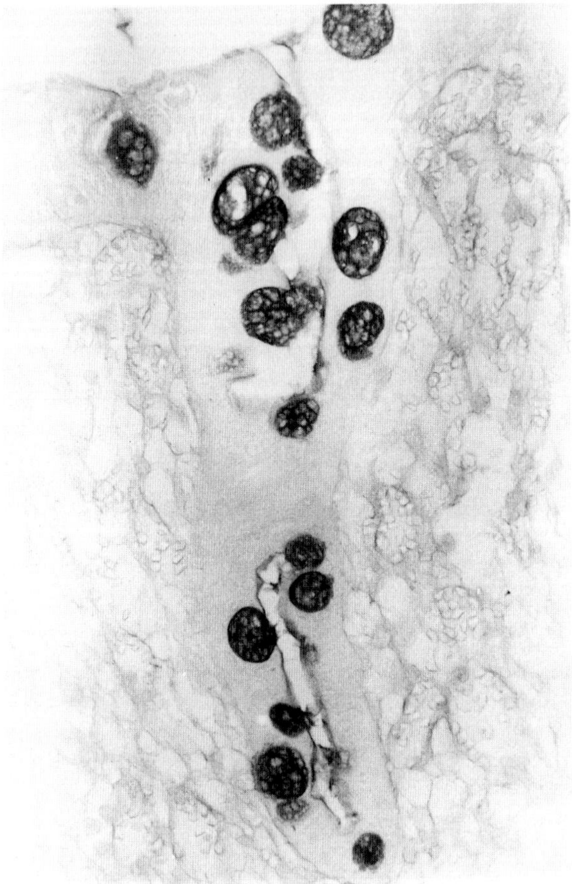

Fig. 2. Complete intestinal metaplasia. Goblet cells stain blue (grey) with high iron diamine/Alcian blue, indicating secretion of nonsulfated acid mucin (sialomucin). Intervening columnar cells do not secrete detectable mucus. High iron diamine/Alcian blue. ×200

intestinal enterocytes are replaced by a population of partially differentiated columnar mucous cells lacking a well developed brush border and the associated brush border enzymes, notably alkaline phosphatase and trehalase [43] (Figs. 3, 4). In addition, Paneth cells are usually absent. Type II IM was divided further into types IIA and IIB according to the mucin histochemistry of the columnar cell population [26]. In IM type IIA the mucins are predominantly of neutral type, though small amounts of sialomucin may be demonstrable. In type IIB the columnar cells secrete mainly sulfomucins. There are no reliable methods of distinguishing type IIA and type IIB other than by the use of mucin histochemistry. Although it has been stated that

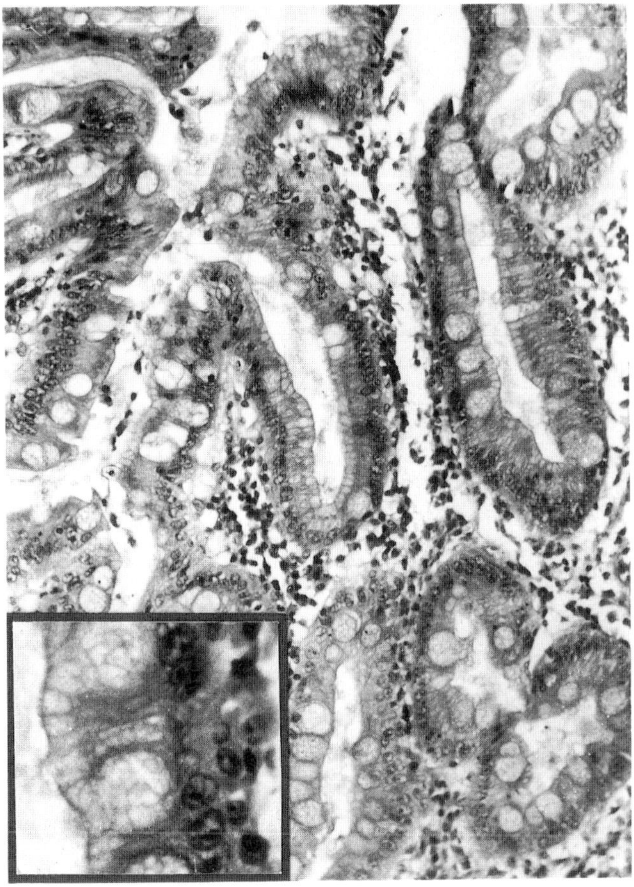

Fig. 3. Incomplete intestinal metaplasia. The epithelium comprises goblet cells and columnar mucous cells. Paneth cells were absent. *Inset* (×300) shows detail of columnar mucous cells which lack a well-developed brush border and contain an apical secretory vesicle. H & E, ×100

type IIB shows more cytological and architectural atypia [75], this is not sufficiently consistent to be diagnostically useful.

It must be admitted that the above classification is an over-simplification. Segura and Montero [74] divided complete IM into two small intestinal types and a colonic type. Ultrastructural studies provide additional insight into the true nature of incomplete IM. Based on light microscopy augmented by mucin histochemistry, incomplete IM appears to be characterized by a combination of goblet cells and columnar mucous cells. However, ultrastructural studies show the columnar cell population to be very much more complex. Levine et al. [40] have demonstrated a "pseudoabsorptive"

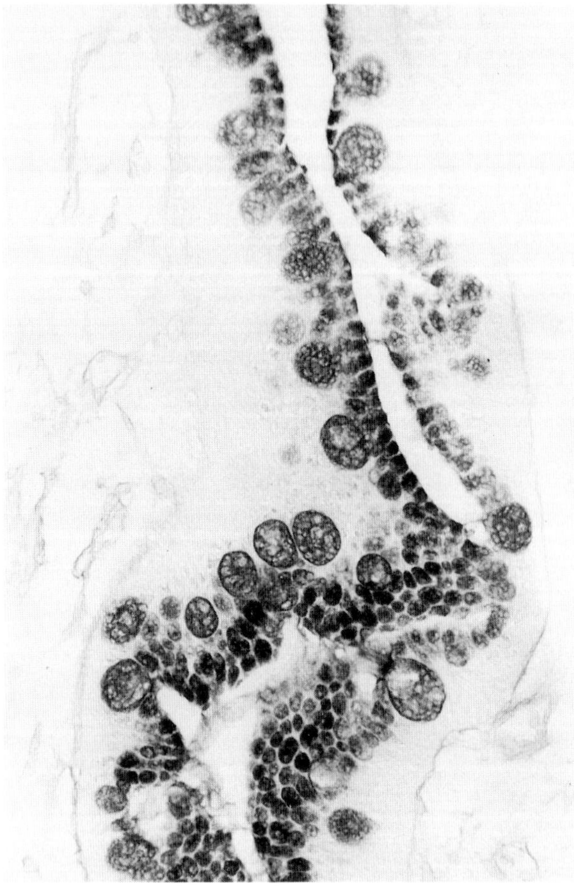

Fig. 4. Incomplete intestinal metaplasia Type IIB. Goblet cells stain blue (grey) with High iron diamine/Alcian blue, indicating secretion of nonsulfated acid mucin (sialomucin). The intervening columnar mucous cells stain dark brown (black) indicating secretion of sulfomucin. This variant of IM is associated with intestinal-type gastric carcinoma. High iron diamine/Alcian blue. ×200

cell and a range of intermediate forms between the pseudoabsorptive cell and typical columnar mucous cells. The pseudoabsorptive cell may have a reasonably well developed brush border and contain little intracytoplasmic mucin. At the light microscope level such cells may easily be misdiagnosed as true absorptive cells, leading to overdiagnosis of complete IM. However, pseudoabsorptive cells always contain small numbers of mucin granules which more closely resemble the droplets of gastric mucous neck cells than gastric crypt and surface columnar mucous cells. In addition, the microvilli vary in size and have a poorly formed terminal web. Other types of columnar cell with features intermediate between metaplastic columnar mucous cells and goblet cells may also be encountered. While columnar in shape, these cells contain mucin droplets with the staining characteristics and ultrastructural appearance of goblet cell mucins. Given these intricacies, the classification of IM by light microscopy and mucin histochemistry clearly falls short of the truth. At this time, however, no-one has succeeded in performing a detailed correlative study of mucin histochemical and ultrastructural features. Despite its shortcomings, the simple classification of IM described at the beginning of this section appears to be of some clinical and epidemiological significance.

Relation Between Variants of IM and Gastric Carcinoma

A considerable number of studies have demonstrated an association between sulfomucin-positive IM and gastric carcinoma. More specifically, this relationship appears to be between type IIB IM (incomplete with sulfomucin production) and intestinal type gastric cancer. These observations have been made in both surgical resection specimens [21, 26, 37, 74, 75, 94] and in endoscopic biopsy material [14, 22, 68, 75, 77]. It should be noted that in one endoscopic biopsy study, type IIB IM was found with high frequency in patients with benign conditions only [55]. This must certainly cast some doubt on the value of type IIB IM as a selective precancerous marker. More importantly, the fortuitous discovery of type IIB IM in a gastric biopsy does not appear to indicate an increased risk of future gastric malignancy [10, 65]. These last studies were retrospective ones, and the results of a large prospective multicenter trial are still awaited [14].

IM in the Lower Esophagus

Intestinalized mucosa may occur in Barrett's esophagus. Although it has been stated that complete IM may occur in this site, an ultrastructural study has shown that true absorptive cells are absent, though "pseudoabsorptive" cells may be seen [40]. These contain small numbers of mucous granules similar to those of mucous neck cells in the stomach. The microvilli vary in length and the terminal webs are poorly formed. In these respects the pseudoabsorptive cells are identical to those occurring in intestinalized gastric mucosa (see above). However, unlike pseudoabsorptive cells of gastric mucosa, the pseudoabsorptive cells in Barrett's esophagus never contain very low density lipoproteins and fail to express brush border hydrolases.

As in incomplete IM of the stomach, the columnar cells within intestinalized Barrett's esophagus may secrete neutral mucin, sialomucin, or sulfomucin [27]. As in gastric incomplete IM, the columnar cell population can be subdivided according to whether or not sulfomucin secretion predominates (as opposed to neutral and/or sialomucins). Sulfomucins are often demonstrated in cardiac-type glands or in the columnar cells of the neck region. Sulfomucin positive variants should only be diagnosed when columnar cells throughout the crypt and surface epithelium give an appropriate staining reaction (e.g., brown with high iron diamine/alcian blue).

The distribution of Barrett's esophagus and histochemical subtypes was studied in 365 patients taking part in a drug trial for reflux esophagitis (Jass et al., unpublished data). Barrett's esophagus was diagnosed histologically in 59 patients (16.2%). Of these, intestinal variants were seen in 27 patients (7.4%), and from this group there were 15 patients (4.1%) with sulfomucin positive columnar cells. No dysplasia was seen. It is of interest that histologically confirmed ulcerative reflux esophagitis mucosa occurred in 51.8% of patients with intestinalized mucosa. Ulcerative reflux esophagitis occurred in only 20.5% of patients without Barrett's esophagus and in 18.7% of patients with columnar epithelium of gastric type. The last may represent inadvertent gastric sampling. This study indicates that intestinalization in the lower esophagus is a marker of severe reflux injury. Furthermore, the data suggest that sulfomucin secretion occurs too frequently to be useful as a selective precancerous marker.

Detailed histological and histochemical studies have demonstrated relationships between intestinalised mucosa of the lower esophagus (especially sulfomucin-positive forms), dysplasia, and adenocarcinoma (Fig. 5). However, it would seem that the neoplastic continuum should be regarded as originating with dysplasia and not at the earlier stage of metaplasia. There is no convincing experimental evidence to support the view that intestinalized mucosa of the lower esophagus amounts to a low grade dysplasia (synonymous with low grade intraepithelial neoplasia). From a more practical standpoint, the high prevalence of sulfomucin-positive IM in Barrett's esophagus is a common sense argument against applying the term dysplasia to this lesion.

The above-mentioned arguments may be extrapolated to the stomach. It is difficult to accept that identical lesions in the lower esophagus and stomach carry different clinical significance. True dysplasia is clinically significant wherever it occurs; it is part of the neoplastic continuum and progression to malignant invasion, and must be regarded as a matter of course in untreated cases. It is therefore unwise to view sulfomucin-positive IM in the stomach as dysplastic (precancerous) when the identical lesion in the lower esophagus is not regarded in this way.

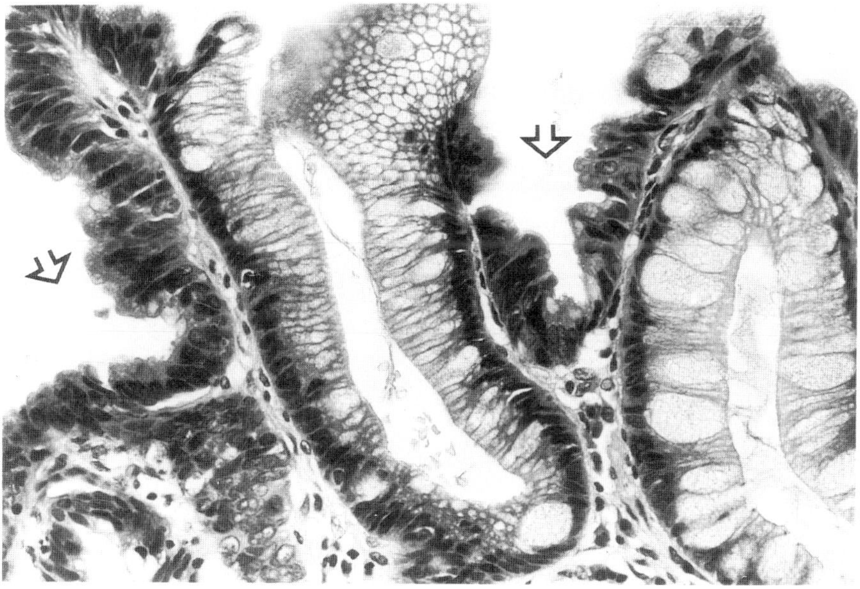

Fig. 5. Dysplasia in Barrett's esophagus. Foci of dysplastic epithelium (*arrows*) are in intimate contact with intestinalized columnar epithelium. The last is similar if not identical to incomplete intestinal metaplasia (IM) of gastric mucosa. Despite the well documented relation between intestinalized (specialized) columnar epithelium, dysplasia and adenocarcinoma of the lower esophagus, the metaplastic change occurs too frequently to serve as a clinically useful risk marker. H & E, ×200

Metaplasia and Abnormal Maturation in the Colon

Altered mucosal differentiation that may be described as "metaplastic" occurs in the colon in a localized form (metaplastic or hyperplastic polyp) and in a diffuse form in ulcerative colitis [28]. The latter represents an interesting analogy to IM as a sequel to chronic atrophic gastritis. Metaplasia of colorectal mucosa in patients with ulcerative colitis is accompanied by a change in the structure and function of columnar cells, namely the conversion of absorptive cells to mucus-secreting cells. The type of mucin secretion is also altered (O-acetylated sialomucin → N-acetylated sialomucin). The change is age-related and more common in the left colon and rectum where colitic injury is likely to be more severe [28]. Histologically, the changes distinctly resemble incomplete IM (Fig. 6). However, metaplasia is a frequent finding in long standing colitis and would not be useful as a precancerous marker. Although the analogy of gastric mucosa with IM must not be taken too far, these comparisons invite general caution when interpretations are offered of the clinical significance of metaplastic-type change in the gastrointestinal tract.

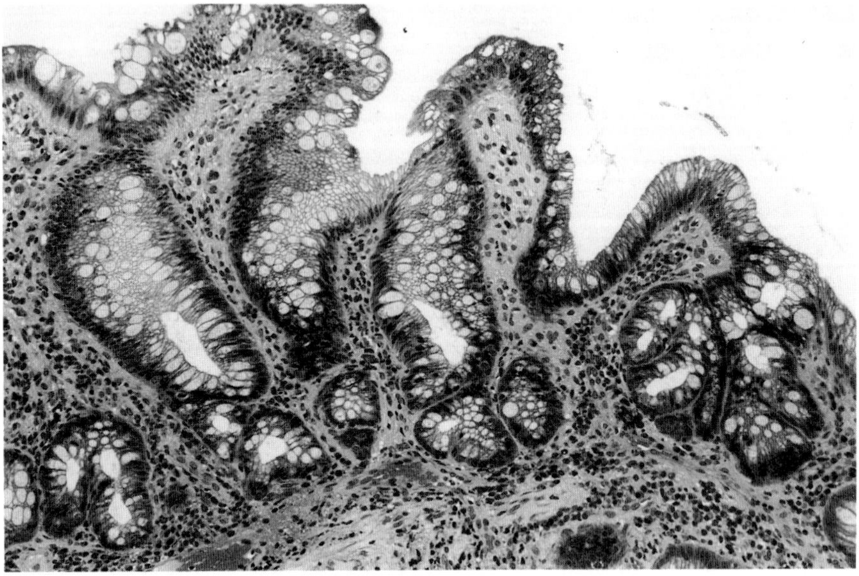

Fig. 6. Incomplete maturation in ulcerative colitis. In addition to the architectural irregularity, careful inspection shows the epithelium to comprise goblet cells and columnar mucous cells. This quite frequent change (metaplasia) is analogous to incomplete IM of stomach and lower esophagus. H & E, ×75

Conclusion

There can be no doubt that an association exists between IM and gastric carcinoma. Indeed, it seems likely that a significant proportion of gastric cancers arise from intestinalized mucosa, particularly intestinal types. However, IM occurs too frequently to serve as a clinically useful risk factor. A more selective association can be demonstrated for variants of IM, notably incomplete forms which secrete sulfomucin (type IIB). The nature and developmental biology of incomplete IM is not yet understood. Similar processes occur in the lower esophagus (Barrett) and in inflammatory bowel disease. Incomplete metaplasia is probably a maturation disturbance and should be distinguished from true dysplasia which is a neoplastic process. In retrospective studies, type IIB IM has not fulfilled its promise as a potential marker of increased cancer risk. Prospective studies are in place, but until the results of these are known there is no justification for following up patients with IM, even if they display the type IIB variant.

References

1. Abe M, Ohuchi N, Sakano H (1974) Enzyme histo and biochemistry of intestinalised gastric mucosa. Acta Histochem Cytochem 7:282–287
2. Borrmann R (1926) Geschwulste des Magens und Duodenums. In: Henke F, Lubarsch (eds) Handbuch der speziellen pathologischen Anatomie und Histologie, vol 4/1. Springer, Berlin, pp 812–1054
3. Burtin P, von Kleist S, Sabine MC, King M (1973) Immunohistological localisation of carcinoembryonic antigen and non-specific cross reacting antigen in gastro-intestinal normal and tumoural tissues. Cancer Res 33:3299–3305
4. Cheng H, Leblond CP (1974) Origin and renewal of the four main epithelial cell types in the mouse small intestine. Am J Anat 141:537–561
5. Correa P (1980) The epidemiology and pathogenesis of chronic gastritis. Three aetiological entities. In: van der Reis L (ed) Frontiers of gastro-intestinal research. Karger, Basel, pp 98–108
6. Correa P, Cuello C, Duque E (1970) Carcinoma and intestinal metaplasia in the stomach of Colombian migrants. JNCI 44:297–306
7. Correa P, Sasano N, Stemmermann GN, Haenszel W (1973) Pathology of gastric carcinoma in Japanese populations: comparisons between Miyagi prefecture, Japan and Hawaii. JNCI 51:1449–1457
8. Cuello C, Correa P, Zarama G, Lopez J, Murray J, Gordillo G (1979) Histopathology of gastric dysplasias. Am J Surg Pathol 3:491–500
9. Culling CFA, Reid PE, Clay MG, Dunn WL (1974) The histochemical demonstration of O-acylated sialic acid in gastro-intestinal mucins: their association with the potassium hydroxide-periodic acid-Schiff effect. Histochem Cytochem 22:826–831
10. Ectors N, Dixon MF (1986) The prognostic value of sulphomucin positive intestinal metaplasia in the development of gastric cancer. Histopathology 10:1271–1277
11. Ejeckam GC, Huang SN, McCaughey WTE, Gold P (1979) Immunohistopathologic study on carcinoembryonic antigen (CEA)-like material and immunoglobulin A in gastric malignancies. Cancer 44:1606–1614
12. Faber K (1935) Gastritis and its consequences. Oxford University Press, New York
13. Fairley KF, Turner CN, MacKay MA, Joske RA (1955) Atrophic gastritis: a five year survey of thirty five cases proven by gastric biopsy. Med J Aust 2:1085–1088
14. Filipe MI, Potet F, Bogomoletz WV, Dawson PA, Fabiani B, Chauveinc P, Fenzy A, Gazzard B, Goldfain D, Zeegen R (1985) Incomplete sulphomucin secreting intestinal metaplasia for gastric cancer. Preliminary data from a prospective study from three centres. Gut 26:1319–1326
15. Gad A (1969) A histochemical study of human alimentary tract mucosubstances in health and disease. I. Normal and tumour. Br J Cancer 23:52–63
16. Glass GBJ, Pitchumoni CS (1975) Atrophic gastritis. Hum Pathol 6:219–250
17. Goldman H, Ming SC (1968) Fine structure of intestinal metaplasia and adenocarcinoma of the human stomach. Lab Invest 18:203–210
18. Goldman H, Ming SC (1968) Mucins in normal and neoplastic gastro-intestinal epithelium. Arch Pathol 85:580–586
19. Guiss LW, Stewart FW (1943) Chronic atrophic gastritis and cancer of the stomach. Arch Surg 46:823–843
20. Hattori T, Fujita S (1979) Tritiated thymidine autoradiographic study on histogenesis and spreading of intestinal metaplasia human stomach. Pathol Res Pract 164:224–237
21. Heilmann KL, Höpker WW (1979) Loss of differentiation in intestinal metaplasia in cancerous stomachs. A comparative morphologic study. Pathol Res Pract 164: 249–258
22. Huang C-B, Xu J, Huang J-F, Meng X-Y (1986) Sulphomucin colonic type intestinal metaplasia and carcinoma in the stomach. Cancer 57:1370–1375
23. Iida F, Murata F, Nagata T (1978) Histochemical studies of mucosubstances in metaplastic epithelium of the stomach with special reference in the development of intestinal metaplasia. Histochem J 56:229–237

24. Imai T, Kubo T, Watanabe H (1971) Chronic gastritis in Japanese with reference to the high incidence of gastric carcinoma. JNCI 47:179–195
25. Järvi O, Laurén P (1951) On the role of heterotopias of the intestinal epithelium in the pathogenesis of gastric carcinoma. Acta Pathol Microbiol Scand 29:26–44
26. Jass JR (1980) Role of intestinal metaplasia in the histogenesis of gastric carcinoma. J Clin Pathol 33:801–810
27. Jass JR (1981) Mucin histochemistry of the columnar epithelium of the oesophagus: a retrospective study. J Clin Pathol 34:866–870
28. Jass JR, Sugihara K, Love SB (1988) Basis of sialic acid heterogeneity in ulcerative colitis. J Clin Pathol 41:388–392
29. Johansen A (1976) Early gastric cancer. In: Morson BC (ed) Current topics in pathology, vol 63. Springer, Berlin Heidelberg New York, pp 1–47
30. Joske RA, Finckh ES, Wood IJ (1955) A study of 1000 consecutive gastric biopsies. Q J Med 24:269–294
31. Kawachi T, Kurisu M, Numanyu N, Sasajima K, Sano T, Sugimura T (1976) Precancerous changes in the stomach. Cancer Res 36:2673–2677
32. Kobori O, Oota K (1974) Mucous substance and enzyme histochemistry of non-neoplastic and neoplastic gastric epithelium in man. Acta Pathol Jpn 24:119–130
33. Konjetzny GE (1938) Der Magenkrebs. Enke, Stuttgart
34. Kupffer C (1883) Epithel and Drüsen des menschlichen Magens. Festschrift des ärtzlichen Vereins München zur Feier seines 50 jährigen Jubiläums, Munich
35. Lambert R (1972) Chronic gastritis. Digestion 7:83–126
36. Laurén P (1965) The two main histological types of gastric carcinoma; diffuse and so-called intestinal type carcinoma. An attempt at a histochemical classification. Acta Pathol Microbiol Scand 64:31–49
37. Lei D-N, Yu J-Y (1984) Types of mucosal metaplasia in relation to the histogenesis of gastric carcinoma. Arch Pathol Lab Med 108:219–224
38. Lev R (1966) The mucin histochemistry of normal and neoplastic gastric mucosa. Lab Invest 14:2080–2100
39. Lev R (1970) The histochemistry of mucus-producing cells in the normal and diseased gastrointestinal mucosa. In: Glass GBJ (ed) Progress in gastroenterology, vol 2. Grune and Stratton, New York, pp 13–41
40. Levine DS, Rubin CE, Reid BJ, Haggitt RC (1989) Specialised metaplastic columnar epithelium in Barrett's esophagus. A comparative transmission electron microscopic study. Lab Invest 60:418–432
41. Ma J, de Boer WGRM, Nayman J (1982) Intestinal mucinous substances in gastric intestinal metaplasia and carcinoma studied by immunofluorescence. Cancer 49: 1664–1667
42. Magnus HA (1937) Observations of the presence of intestinal epithelium in the gastric mucosa. J Pathol Bacteriol 44:389–397
43. Matsukura N, Suzuki K, Kawachi T, Aoyagi M, Sugimura T, Kitaoka H, Numajiri H, Shirota A, Itabashi M, Hirota T (1980) Distribution of marker enzymes and mucin in intestinal metaplasia in human stomachs and relation of complete and incomplete types of intestinal metaplasia to minute gastric carcinomas. JNCI 65:231–240
44. Ming SC (1979) Dysplasia of gastric epithelium. Front Gastrointest Res 4:164–172
45. Ming SC, Goldman H, Freiman DG (1967) Intestinal metaplasia and histogenesis of carcinoma of the human stomach. Cancer 20:1418–1429
46. Morson BC (1955) Intestinal metaplasia of the gastric mucosa. Br J Cancer 9:365–376
47. Morson BC (1955) Carcinoma arising from areas of intestinal metaplasia in the gastric mucosa. Br J Cancer 9:377–385
48. Morson BC, Sobin LM, Grundmann E, Johansen A, Nagayo T, Serck-Mansen A (1980) Precancerous conditions and epithelial dysplasia in the stomach. J Clin Pathol 33:711–721
49. Motteram RA (1951) A biopsy study of chronic gastritis and gastric atrophy. J Pathol Bacteriol 63:389–394
50. Mukawa K, Nakamura T, Nakano G, Nagamachi Y (1987) Histopathogenesis of intestinal metaplasia: minute lesions of intestinal metaplasia in ulcerated stomachs. J Clin Pathol 40:13–18

51. Mulligan RM, Rember RR (1954) Histogenesis and biologic behaviour of gastric carcinoma. Arch Pathol 58:1–25
52. Muñoz N, Asvall J (1971) Time trends of intestinal and diffuse types of gastric cancer in Norway. Int J Cancer 8:144–157
53. Muñoz N, Matko I (1972) Histological types of gastric cancer and its relationships with intestinal metaplasia. In: Grundmann E, Tulinius H (eds) Current problems in the epidemiology of cancer and lymphomas. Springer, Berlin Heidelberg New York, pp 99–105 (Recent results in cancer research, vol 39)
54. Muñoz N, Correa P, Cuello C, Duque E (1968) Histologic types of gastric carcinoma in high and low risk areas. Int J Cancer 3:809–818
55. Murray LA, Williams GT (1984) Sulphomucin containing intestinal metaplasia in gastric biopsies – one year's experience. J Pathol 142:A24
56. Nagayo T (1971) Histological diagnosis of biopsied gastric mucosa with special reference to that of borderline lesions. Gann Monogr Cancer Res 11:245–256
57. Nagayo T (1981) Dysplasia of the gastric mucosa and its relation to the precancerous state. Gan 72:813–823
58. Nakahara K (1978) Special features of intestinal metaplasia and its relation to early gastric carcinoma in man: observation by a method in which leucine aminopeptidase activity is used. JNCI 61:693–701
59. Nakamura K, Sugano H, Takagi K (1968) Carcinoma of the stomach in incipient phase; its histogenesis and histological appearances. Gan 59:251–258
60. Nevalainen TJ, Järvi OH (1977) Ultrastructure of intestinal and diffuse type gastric carcinoma. J Pathol 122:129–136
61. Oehlert W, Keller P, Henke M, Strauch M (1979) Gastric mucosal dysplasia: what is their clinical significance? Front Gastroint Res 4:173–182
62. Oohara T, Tohma H, Takezoe K, Ukawa S, Johjima Y, Asakura R, Aono G, Kurosaka H (1982) Minute gastric cancers less than 5 mm in diameter. Cancer 50: 801–810
63. Oohara T, Tohma H, Aono G, Ukawa S, Knodo Y (1983) Intestinal metaplasia of the regenerative epithelium in 549 gastric ulcers. Hum Pathol 14:1066–1071
64. Planteydt HT, Willighagen RGJ (1960) Enzyme histochemistry of the human stomach with special reference to intestinal metaplasia. J Pathol Bacteriol 80:317–322
65. Ramesar KCRB, Sanders DSA, Hopwood D (1987) Limited value of type III intestinal metaplasia in predicting risk of gastric carcinoma. J Clin Pathol 40: 1287–1290
66. Rapp W, Windisch M, Peschke P, Wurster K (1979) Purification of human intestinal goblet cell antigen (GOA), its immunological demonstration in the intestine and in mucus producing gastrointestinal adenocarcinomas. Virchows Arch [Pathol Anat] 382:163–177
67. Reynolds KW, Johnson AG, Fox BC (1975) Is intestinal metaplasia of the gastric mucosa a premalignant lesion? Oncology 1:101–109
68. Rothery GA, Day DW (1985) Intestinal metaplasia in endoscopic biopsy specimens of gastric mucosa. J Clin Pathol 38:613–621
69. Rubin W, Ross RH, Jeffries GH, Sleisinger MH (1966) Intestinal heterotopia – a fine structural study. Lab Invest 15:1024–1049
70. Rubin W, Ross LL, Sleisenger MH, Jeffries GH (1968) The normal human gastric epithelia. A fine structural study. Lab Invest 19:598–628
71. Sasano N, Nakamura K, Arai M, Akazaki K (1969) Ultrastructural cell patterns in human gastric carcinoma compared with non-neoplastic gastric mucosa-histogenetic analysis of carcinoma by mucin histochemistry. JNCI 43:783–802
72. Schade ROK (1974) The borderline between benign and malignant lesion in the stomach. In: Grundmann E, Gruntze H, Witte S (eds) Early gastric cancer. Springer, Berlin Heidelbeg New York, pp 45–53
73. Schmidt A (1896) Untersuchungen über das menschliche Magenepithel unter normalen und pathologischen Verhältnissen. Virchows Arch [Pathol Anat] 143: 477–508
74. Segura DI, Montero C (1983) Histochemical characterization of different types of intestinal metaplasia in gastric mucosa. Cancer 52:498–503

75. Silva S, Filipe MI (1986) Intestinal metaplasia and its variants in the gastric mucosa of Portuguese subjects: a comparative analysis of biopsy and gastrectomy material. Hum Pathol 17:988–995
76. Sipponen P, Siurala M (1977) Immunological aspects in screening for gastric carcinoma. In: Varro V, Balint GA (eds) Current views in gastroenterology. Hungarian Society of Gastroenterology, Budapest, pp 527–529
77. Sipponen P, Seppälä K, Varis K, Hjelt L, Ihamäki T, Kekki M, Siurala M (1980) Intestinal metaplasia with colonic-type sulphomucins in the gastric mucosa, its association with gastric carcinoma. Acta Pathol Microbiol Scand 88:217–224
78. Sipponen P, Kekki M, Siurala M (1983) Atrophic chronic gastritis and intestinal metaplasia in gastric carcinoma. Comparison with a representative population sample. Cancer 52:1062–1068
79. Siurala M, Seppälä K (1960) Atrophic gastritis as a possible precursor of gastric carcinoma and pernicious anaemia. Acta Med Scand 166:455–474
80. Siurala M, Isokoski M, Varis K, Kekki M (1968) Prevalence of gastritis in a rural population. Bioptic study of subjects selected at random. Scand J Gastroenterol 3:211–223
81. Skinner JM, Heenan PJ, Whitehead R (1975) Atrophic gastritis in gastrectomy specimens. Br J Surg 62:23–25
82. Slack JMW (1985) Homoeotic transformations in man: implications for the mechanism of embryonic development and for the organisation of epithelia. J Theor Biol 114:463–490
83. Stemmermann GN (1967) Comparative study of histochemical patterns in non-neoplastic and neoplastic gastric epithelium. A study of Japanese in Hawaii. JNCI 39:375–383
84. Stemmermann GN, Hayashi T (1968) Intestinal metaplasia of the gastric mucosa: a gross and microscopic study of its distribution in various disease states. JNCI 41: 627–634
85. Stockton M, McColl I (1983) Comparative electron microscopic features of normal, intermediate and metaplastic pyloric epithelium. Histopathology 7:859–871
86. Stoffels GL, Desnaux JJ, Gepts W (1972) Gastroscopic and histochemical study of normal, atrophic and hypertrophic mucosa. Digestion 6:23–34
87. Stout AP (1953) In: Atlas of tumour pathology, vol 6. Armed Forces Institute of Pathology, Washington
88. Tarpila S, Telkkä A, Siurala M (1969) Ultrastructure of various metaplasias of the stomach. Acta Pathol Microbiol Scand 77:187–195
89. Taylor AL, (1927) The epithelial heterotopias of the alimentary tract. J Pathol Bacteriol 30:415–449
90. Teglbjaerg PS, Nielsen HO (1978) "Small intestinal type" and "colonic type" intestinal metaplasia of the human stomach. Acta Pathol Microbiol Scand 86:351–355
91. Walker IR, Strickland IG, Ungar B, Mackay IR (1971) Simple atrophic gastritis and gastric carcinoma. Gut 12:906–911
92. Warren S, Meissner WA (1944) Chronic gastritis and carcinoma of the stomach. Gastroenterology 3:251–256
93. Wattenberg LW (1959) Histochemical study of aminopeptidase in metaplasia and carcinoma of the stomach. Arch Pathol 67:281–286
94. Wells M, Stewart M, Dixon MF (1982) Mucin histochemistry of gastric intestinal metaplasia. J Pathol 138:70
95. Whitehead R, Truelove SC, Gear MWL (1972) The histological diagnosis of chronic gastritis in fibreoptic gastroscope biopsy specimens. J Clin Pathol 25:1–11
96. Wood IJ, Taft LI (1958) Diffuse lesions of the stomach. Arnold, London
97. Wyatt JI, Dixon MF (1988) Chronic gastritis – a pathogenetic approach. J Pathol 154:113–124

6 Typing and Grading of Gastric Dysplasia

Y.-C. Zhang

Introduction

Most pathologists agree that gastric dysplasia, or epithelial dysplasia of the stomach, is an important precancerous change within the stomach. There is, however, much confusion about the nomenclature to be used for such changes. The term "gastric dysplasia" was proposed by a WHO Workshop on Histological Criteria of Precancerous Change of the Stomach in 1978, and it has since been used widely by pathologists [3, 5, 18–21, 27, 32, 38, 45].

Other terms, such as "atypical epithelial lesion" (ATP) [6, 24, 28, 31] and subtype IIa, have been described in the literature. But ATP is not a synonym for gastric dysplasia as the latter has a wider scope or includes a range of histopathologic changes. In other words, ATP is merely one kind of gastric dysplasia.

The term "borderline lesion of the stomach", proposed by Nagayo [22], has also been found in the literature. It is another name for ATP and as Group III of the classification for mucosal biopsy materials, cited in The General Rules for Gastric Cancer Study, published by the Japanese Research Society for Gastric Cancer [7].

Increases in our understanding of the importance of gastric dysplasia have depended upon improvements in examination techniques for gastric diseases; more studies have been made of early gastric carcinomas, especially microcarcinomas, and more emphasis placed on the discovery of lesions related to the histogenesis of gastric carcinoma, including the clinical cases, and also on animal experiments concerning the induction of gastric cancer. Yet many things about gastric dysplasia remain unclear, specifically the histogenesis or the relationship between the types of gastric dysplasias and the respective histopathologic types of gastric carcinoma and also the objective criteria of the malignant potentials or degrees of atypia for a given case of gastric dysplasia.

Cancer Institute of China Medical University, 5-3 Nanjing Street, Heping District, Shenyang, P.R. China

Ying-Chan Zhang/Keiichi Kawai (Eds.)
Precancerous Conditions and Lesions of the Stomach

There are different views, too, about biological behavior. Gastric dysplasia is looked upon as an academic term signifying an abnormality which should be identifiable, if present, in a mucosal biopsied specimen. But it is often difficult to come to a clear decision. In the matters of deciding whether a lesion is irreversible or not, and what suggestions should be made to clinicians while pathologists seek to detect the dysplastic lesion in the biopsied specimen, different pathologists often develop different views and opinions, many of which are based on their own experiences. All these problems stem from a lack of clear and accurate guidelines and explicit knowledge. Further study is therefore well merited.

Histopathology of Gastric Dysplasia

Gastric dysplasia is a histopathological concept. Whether it be studied in the form of surgically resected specimens or mucosal biopsy material, a great deal of understanding is required if this kind of pathological change is to be correctly interpreted, typed and graded. Gastric dysplasia implies two things: (a) disorganized mucosal glandular architecture, such as glandular spare or dense or tortuous misshape, and (b) disorganized arrangement. Back-to-back arrangement of the glandular tubules, budding, branching or interanastomosis of the tubules and sometimes papillary growth have usually been seen.

Cellular changes include atypia and abnormal differentiation of the epithelial cells. Features of these changes are nuclear pleomorphism, hyperchromatism, and an increased ratio of nucleus to cytoplasm, though the nuclear arrangement of gastric dysplasia is mostly localized at the base of the cells. The effect is of cells which are somewhat disorganized and closely packed together in varying degrees. In severe cases, loss of polarity occurs. Another cytological change is abnormal cellular differentiation. In the intestinal type of dysplasia, goblet cells and Paneth cells decrease or disappear. The component of mucus is also usually changed.

Studies conducted in the last twenty years have persuaded us that it is necessary to produce a rational typing or classification for working out objective criteria for evaluating degrees of dysplasia. Different types of gastric dysplasia have their own pathogenesis and developing patterns. If dysplasias of different histogenetic types are compared, with a view to assessing degrees of dysplasia and potential malignancy, then unified, accurate judging criteria will certainly not be obtained [38, 40]. Although many pathologists have produced different classifications of gastric dysplasia over the years [3, 10, 38], we consider that the typing suggested in the following paragraph might now be appropriate.

Repeated comparison and analysis of specimens of gastric dysplasia from more than 300 cases have been made and five types of gastric dysplasia are proposed:

1. Cryptal
2. Adenomatous
3. Regenerative
4. Globoid
5. Cystic

Cryptal and adenomatous dysplasias consist of intestinal epithelia, but their histogenesis and characteristics differ from each other. As for regenerative and globoid dysplasias, both consist of gastric and intestinal type epithelium. We believe that this typing can more exactly reflect the characteristics and developing tendencies of gastric dysplasias.

Cryptal Dysplasia

Cryptal dysplasia is a common type of gastric dysplasia which occurs mainly in the deeper portion of intestinal metaplastic mucosa, i.e., it originates from the crypts of metaplastic glands, especially in severe chronic atrophic or atrophic-hyperplastic gastritis. Because the dysplastic change occurs at the base of intestinal metaplastic glands, the dysplasia often retains some features of intestinal epithelium. Some of the type IIB intestinal metaplasias of Jass (see Chap. 5, "classification of IM") may be responsible for this type of gastric dysplasia [17, 21]. Columnar cells with brush border are the main forming cells while goblet cells and Paneth cells usually decrease or disappear.

Mild. In general, mild cryptal dysplasia can be distinguished as emergence during the extension from the metaplastic tubule towards the deeper portion of the mucosa. The dysplastic tubule shows mild tortuosity. Its size and shape more or less keep the original features of intestinal metaplastic glands. Goblet cells decrease, or only their vestiges remain; therefore, they mostly consist of columnar epithelia with brush border. The nuclei become rod-shaped and closely crowded at the basal portion of cells; their arrangement is ordered. Mitotic figures are seldom seen, while Paneth cells disappear. The dysplastic tubules form many clusters but without a clear borderline.

Moderate. The glands of moderate cryptal dysplasia show crowded focus of dysplastic tubules. These tubules are irregular in size and shape. All the epithelial cells are high columnar. Arrangement of the nuclei shows varying degrees of disorder.

Severe. In severe cryptal dysplasia, many dysplastic tubules are to be seen crowded into clusters or foci. Size and shape of the dysplasia are irregular; moreover, dilated tubules are often seen to be forming cysts. The dysplastic epithelium shows high columnar form while the brush borders are not sure to be clear. The nuclei become long-rod-shaped, hyperchromatized and

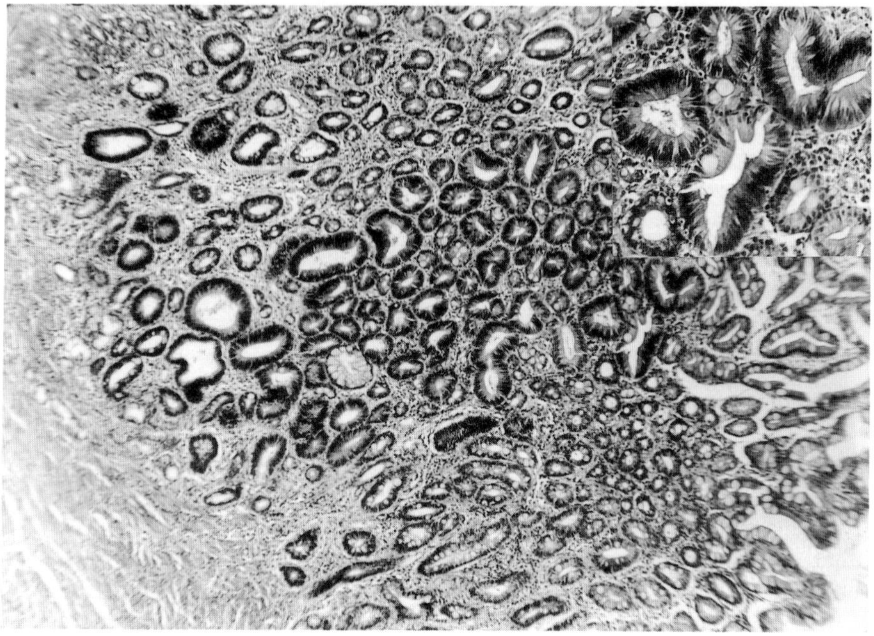

Fig. 1. Cryptal dysplasia. The dysplasia is seen in the deep portion of the gastric mucosa. The dysplastic tubules are mingling with intestinal metaplastic tubules and there is no marked borderline between these and the dysplastic focus with its surrounding tissue. H & E, ×80.

disordered in arrangement. Mitotic figures can be detected. The dysplastic focus is adenoma-like, but usually there is no clear demarcation between the dysplastic focus and its surrounding intestinal metaplastic glands. It is here that the difference between cryptal dysplasia and adenomatous dysplasia is seen (Fig. 1).

Adenomatous Dysplasia

Most of the adenomatous dysplasias have protruding foci. Many authors have called these dysplasias flat adenomas. Japanese pathologists usually named this type of dysplasia "atypical epithelial lesion" (ATP) [25, 29] or subtype IIa [4]; the dysplasia consists of crowded dysplastic tubules. The size and shape of the tubules are irregular, even pseudopapillary. The focus has clear demarcation from its surrounding tissue and, usually, there is no obvious pressing of the focus against the latter. In the deeper portion of the focus, it is common to find cystic dilatations of the tubules. Epithelium of adenomatous dysplasia is of a columnar intestinal metaplastic type. Some-

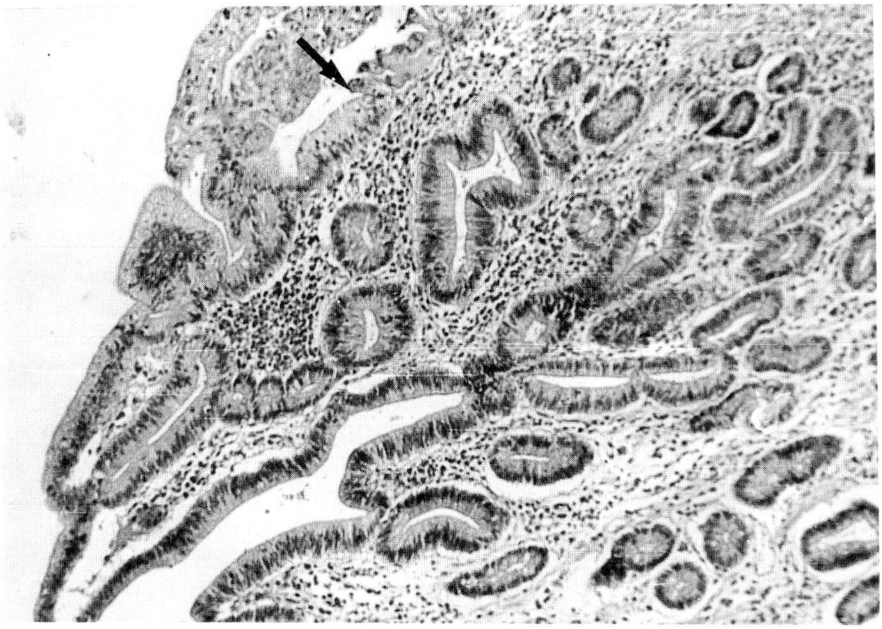

Fig. 2. Adenomatous dysplasia of moderate degree but in which there is malignant transformation. The *arrow* indicates the transitional portion of malignant change. The dysplastic focus is located in the superficial portion of the gastric mucosa. Its epithelial cells show columnar shape with rod-shaped and hyperstained nuclei arranged mostly in the basal portion of the dysplastic epithelia. H & E, ×80

times, in the apex cytoplasm, mucous granules can be detected. The nuclei, which are of a long-rod form, show hyperchromatism and a moderate degree of atypia (Fig. 2), whereas in severe cases the dysplastic epithelium is usually irregular in shape with unclear brush borders. The arrangement of nuclei is uniform. In mucin stain sections sialomucins and sulfomucins (besides traces of neutral mucin), are the main secretions, but in severe cases mucins only can be detected on the free border of the dysplastic epithelium [39].

Although both adenomatous and cryptal dysplasias consist of intestinal epithelium, the former starts from the superficial portion of gastric mucosa and involves only one-third or one-half or two-thirds or almost the whole layer of the mucosa, while the cryptal dysplasias originate from the deeper layer of the mucosa, i.e., the crypts of intestinal metaplastic glands. The characteristics and histogenesis of the two dysplasias differ from each other and we are convinced that adenomatous dysplasia is neoplastic in nature. Adenomatous dysplasias are usually protruding in shape but occasionally show depressed focus [26]. In the five groups for grading of mucosal biopsy proposed by the Japanese Research Society for Gastric Cancer, this type of dysplasia is listed in Group III and named "border line lesion".

Regenerative Dysplasia

In the study of gastric dysplasias, those which occur during the process of gastric mucosal regeneration have generally received far less attention than cryptal and especially adenomatous dysplasias. Indeed, it has even been suspected that regenerative dysplasias may not be precancerous in nature. Regeneration of gastric mucosa is a common phenomenon. Some lesions, certainly, are very slight or limited to superficial epithelial exfoliations or superficial mucosal defects; some others, however are subject to severe repeated erosions and repairing processes. It was believed that most chronic gastritis occurred on the basis of gastric mucosal damages and defects. Through studying a large number of specimens, we found that many "twinkling scenes" (which we shall describe later) at the start point of malignant change occurred in regenerating gastric glands or tubules with dysplasia.

In some of our cases we detected erosions and regenerations of gastric mucosa, and also malignant changes in regenerative dysplasia. A geographic factor may well be at work here because it was found in a mass survey for gastric cancer in Northern China (Liaoning Province), that erosions and regenerations accompanying chronic gastritis were much more common than in Japan even though both areas are areas of similarly high risk [44].

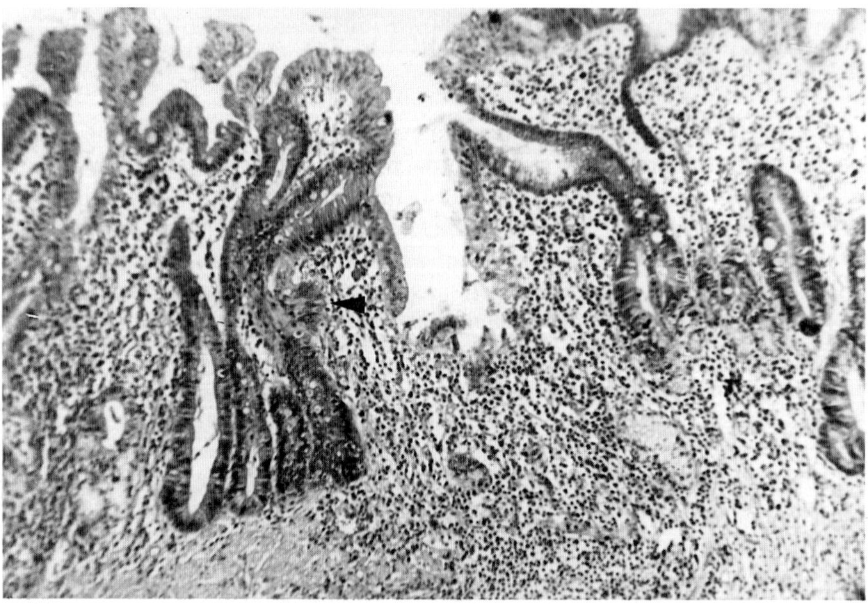

Fig. 3. A clump of "dysplastic epithelia" is penetrating the basement membrane of the regenerating gastric tubule into the lamina propria (*arrow*) while on its right side, a focus of erosion remains. H & E, ×80

The regenerative dysplastic epithelia may be gastric or intestinal; neither of them has any secretory function, and they have no typical architectures due to dedifferentiation. Some of the regenerative dysplastic mucosae are rather thin because of severe damage and for repairing processes. The regenerated glands are spare and irregular; in fact, there are glandular fissures which make the surface of the mucosa rather rough. In a few cases, the pyloric glands or preexisting intestinal metaplastic glands remain. Many features of malignant change were detected. Usually, in the neck zone of regenerated tubules, a cluster of malignant transformed "dysplastic" epithelial cells just blocking and penetrating the basement membrane and infiltrating the stroma was found (Figs. 3, 4). There are the twinkling scenes at the start point, or the microscopic incipient cancer foci, of malignant change in regenerative dysplasia (Figs. 5, 6).

In slightly more advanced cases, the malignant, transformed "dysplastic" epithelial cells infiltrate the stroma in the form of many branches or narrow strands or networks (Fig. 7). In immunohistochemical staining, these cells were strongly positive for carcinoembryonic antigen (CEA) and also showed loss of polarity of the distribution of CEA within the cells.

In some cases, the malignant characteristics of the dysplastic epithelial cells were striking, i.e., basophilia of cytoplasm, enlarged and irregular nuclei, hyperchromatism, and loss of polarity could all be seen; their malig-

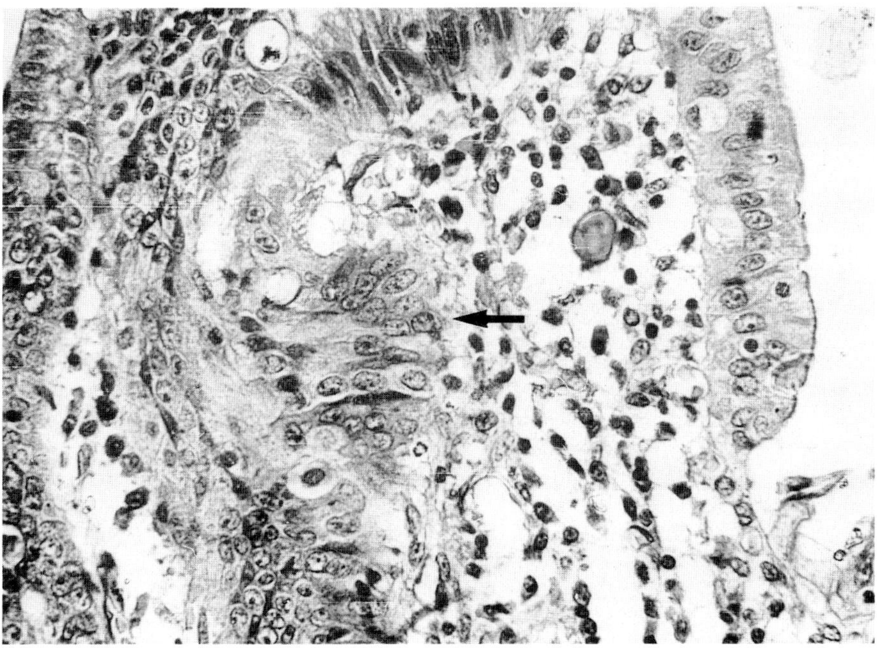

Fig. 4. An enlarged view of the start point (*arrow*) of malignant change shown in Fig. 3. H & E, ×320

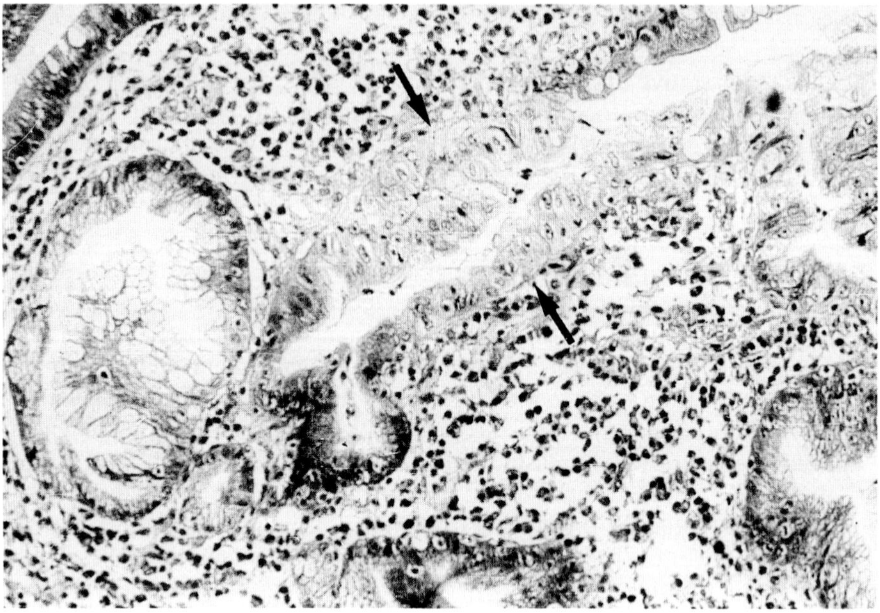

Fig. 5. Malignant change in the neck zone of a regenerated gastric tubule (*arrow*). The "dysplastic" epithelia are penetrating the basement membrane of the tubule and infiltrating the lamina propria. H & E, ×250

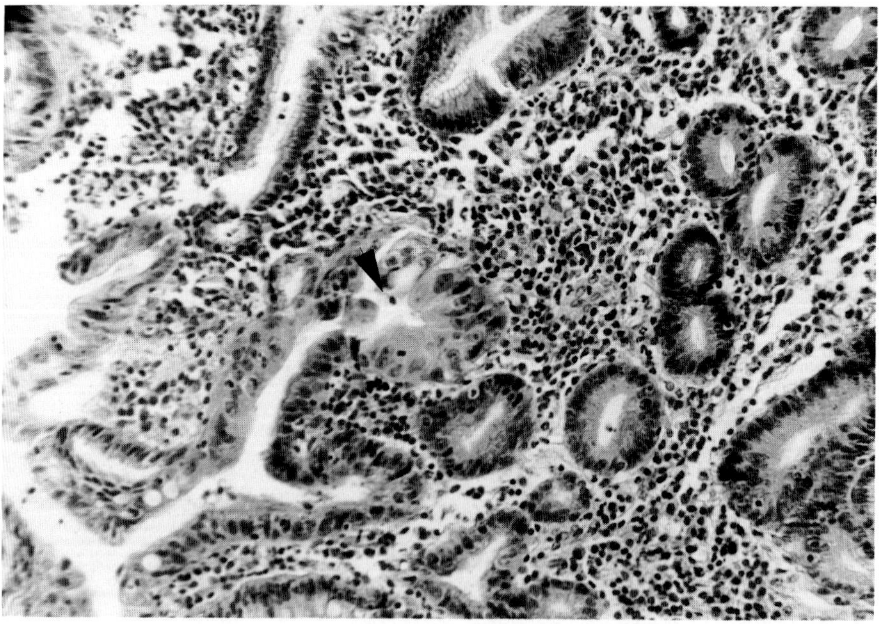

Fig. 6. Regenerated gastric tubule. At the neck zone of the tubule a start point of malignant transformation is visible (*arrow*). H & E, ×250

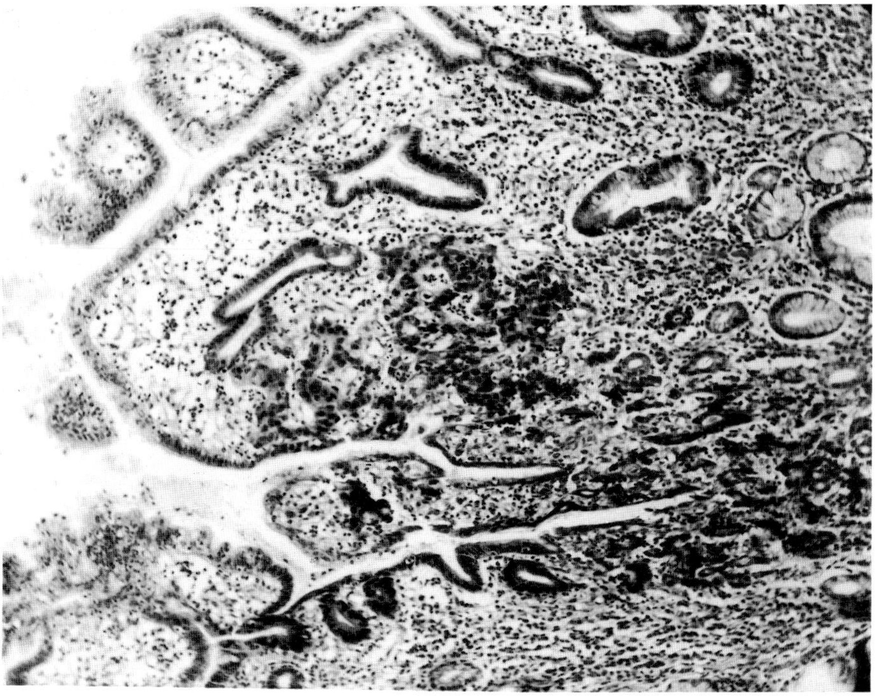

Fig. 7. From the foveola of regenerated gastric mucosa. Many "dysplastic" epithelial cells are infiltrating the stroma and forming many branches and strands. H & E, ×80

nancy, however, was uncertain because these cells were still arranging themselves within the regenerated tubules.

Globoid Dysplasia

Globoid dysplasia has been described as a precancerous lesion in recent years [1, 2], and I have been involved in precise studies of this dysplasia [13–17]. We found that in mucosal biopsies and surgically resected stomach specimens from the human stomach globoid dysplasia usually accompanied diffuse type gastric cancer, particularly signet-ring cell carcinomas. Furthermore, in 53 of our cases in which globoid dysplasia was found to accompany signet-ring cell carcinoma, we found many of the severe grade globoid cells penetrating the basement membrane and infiltrating the stroma. We also noted the formation of incipient foci of signet-ring cell carcinomas.

Globoid dysplasias were grouped into two histopathologic types: (a) type I globoid dysplasia, originating from the D (dissociated) type cell, and (b) type II, which usually occurred in incomplete intestinal metaplasia [14–17].

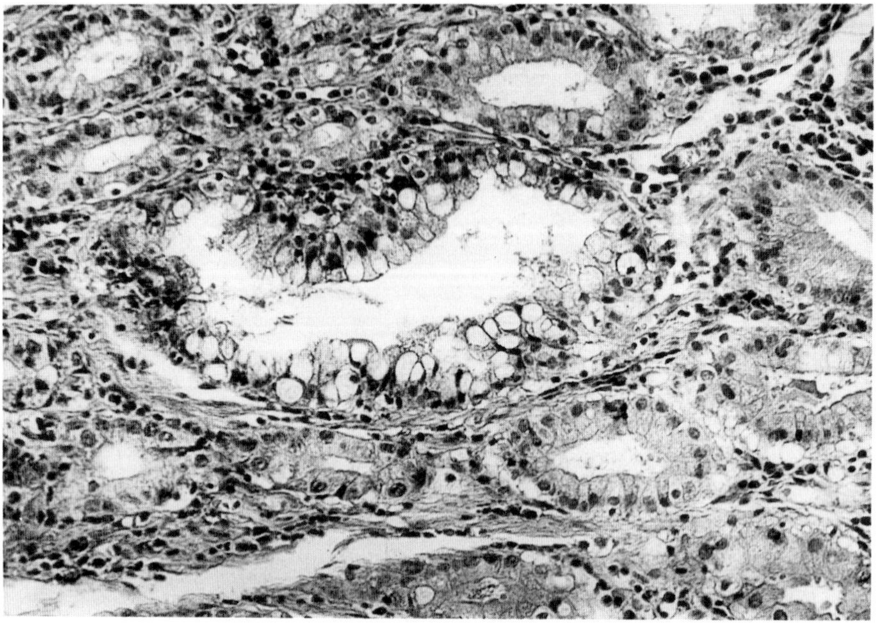

Fig. 8. Globoid dysplasia is detected in the neck zone of a pyloric gland in a resected stomach specimen bearing signet-ring cell carcinoma. Globoid cells became crowded with mucus and showed loss of polarity. H & E, ×300

Globoid cells of these two types were round or oval in shape, their cytoplasm contents neutral, sialo-, and/or sulfomucin. The nucleus of each cell was located in one side, hyperstained, and semilunar in shape. Sometimes, nucleoli were clearly seen. The globoid cells were usually detected in the mucous neck zone or crypts of intestinal metaplastic glands. No matter whether the globoid cells were single or in a cluster, their pecularity was loss of polarity (Fig. 8). According to their architectural and cellular atypia, globoid dysplasias were divided into three grades [13].

Grade I: The globoid cells appeared singly or in a cluster, even occupying a segment of the tubule. The cells were irregular in arrangement but polarity was preserved.

Grade II: There was an obvious increase of mucus in the globoid cells. Loss of polarity appeared even to be reversed. The cells showed up as a cluster in the tubule and the basement membrane was intact.

Grade III: The findings of Grade II were apparent. In addition, the globoid cells were found to be moving to the basement membrane; microscopically, their shape was difficult to differentiate from that of the signet-ring cell [16]. Sometimes, a double layer structure appeared, i.e., the epithelial cells (gastric or metaplastic) facing the lumen preserved its normal shape but the globoid cells were located on the outside (Fig. 9). In such

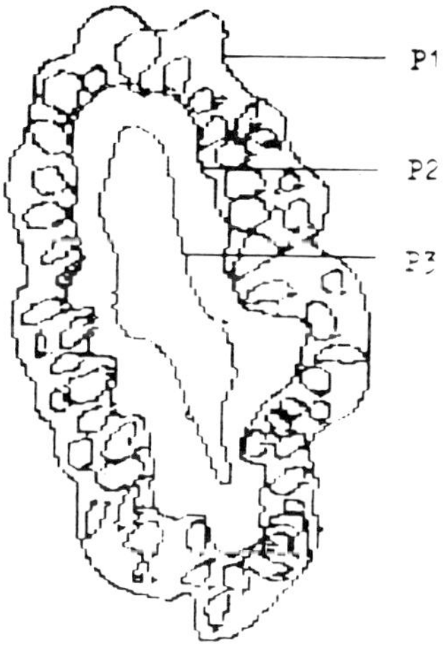

Fig. 9. Typed figure of a dysplastic tubule from the Autoimage Analysis System shows the measurements of P1, P2, and P3

cases, the basement membrane was usually incomplete on Gordon Sweet staining. These findings coincide with those found in the specimens of ENNG-induced signet-ring cell carcinoma in wolf dogs [35].

In analyzing the age and sex distributions of patients with globoid dysplasia and signet-ring cell carcinoma, it was found that the average age of females with these two diseases was 10 years younger than that of males. Generally, the average age of females with signet-ring cell carcinoma and globoid dysplasia was 15 years younger than that of those with well differentiated adenocarcinoma [13].

Cystic Dysplasia

In recent years, dysplastic cysts or cystic dysplasias have been reported by many pathologists. The histopathological characteristics of these cysts are such that they exist singularly or in clusters of varying size with the same dysplastic epithelium as that discovered in gastric mucosa but without other dysplastic focus. Usually, degenerated or necrotic cells, or their debris, were found in these cysts. Retrospective and follow-up studies have verified that these cysts are usually accompanied by early gastric cancer, mostly small cancer or microcancer. It is important to bear in mind that, in the author's follow-up study of 15 patients with intramucosal dysplastic cysts, there were six cases in which early gastric cancer occurred and, among these, three were identified within 3 months to 1 year as small cancer. It is stressed that, because the period of time from discovery of the dysplastic cysts to the occurrence of early cancer was rather short, these kinds of cysts can be said to be close to being antecedents of malignant change [12]. Li et al. [12] also pointed out that these kinds of dysplastic cysts are not the same as the intramucosal cysts accompanying protruded adenomatous dysplasias or atypical epithelial lesions.

Grading of Gastric Dysplasia

Grading of gastric dysplasia owes much to the particular person carrying out the grading. The architectural and cellular atypia exists in a state of transitional change. The frankly benign and malignant changes are easily judged. But it is very difficult to grade degrees of dysplastia within a range of lesions which exhibit less clear-cut atypia. For convenience in practice, it is necessary to divide gastric dysplasias into the three grades mentioned below.

Mild Dysplasia

The mucosal architecture and epithelial cells in mild dysplasia show slight atypia and are certainly benign lesions.

The glandular structures are tortuous and irregular in shape. The dysplastic changes are limited to the superficial or deeper portion of the mucosa. Mucinous secretions are still preserved in mild gastric type dysplasia, while in mild intestinal type dysplasia goblet cells and Paneth cells are decreased. In both types of dysplasia, the nuclei are slightly enlarged or still retain their normal shape.

Moderate Dysplasia

The mucosal architecture and epithelial cells in moderate dysplasia are also benign, but they show frank atypia. The glandular tubules become irregular in size and shape, and are usually packed together. "Budding" and branching of tubules are common. The dysplastic focus is clearly seen histologically. Its epithelium shows high columnar shape with rod-shaped, hyperstained nucleus packed tightly in the basal portion in the cell but somewhat irregular in its arrangement. Most of the Group III or borderline lesions are consistent with this grade of dysplasia.

Severe Dysplasia

In severe gastric dysplasia, glandular architecture is disorganized, its sizes and shapes varying in an obvious way. Besides "budding" and branching of the tubules, back-to-back phenomena of the dysplastic tubules are usually seen. The morphology of dysplastic epithelium is rather important for evaluating the degree of atypia. In severe dysplasia the epithelial cells are also high columnar in shape but somewhat uneven. The nucleus/cytoplasm ratio becomes larger and its arrangement is irregular. Mitotic figures can be seen while mucous secretion disappears.

In the opinion of many pathologists, mild gastric dysplasias is of no clinical importance, i.e., not precancerous in nature. It has also been proposed, therefore, by the Chinese Cooperative Study Group on Gastric Cancer Pathology, that it is not necessary to dagnose this dysplasia as a precancerous lesion. The International Study Group on Gastric Cancer (San Miniato, Italy 1982), has also stressed that mild gastric dysplasia is an atypical hyperplasia but not a precancerous lesion.

Morphometric Indexes for Grading of Gastric Dysplasia

Until now, judgement of dysplastic severity or degrees of atypia in gastric dysplasia has often depended on the pathologist's own experience and has usually been influenced by subjective factors. In recent years, in order to minimise subjective interpretation, morphometric studies have been carried out. Autoimage analysis systems have been used by many pathologists to evaluate degrees of dysplastic change [8, 11, 34, 36, 37, 46].

Taking into account both architectural and cellular atypia, we have proposed N/C, P1/D1, P2/D2 as the objective indexes for evaluating gastric dysplasias [34, 36, 37].

The measurements and calculations from the autoimage analysis system are as follows (Figs. 9 and 10):

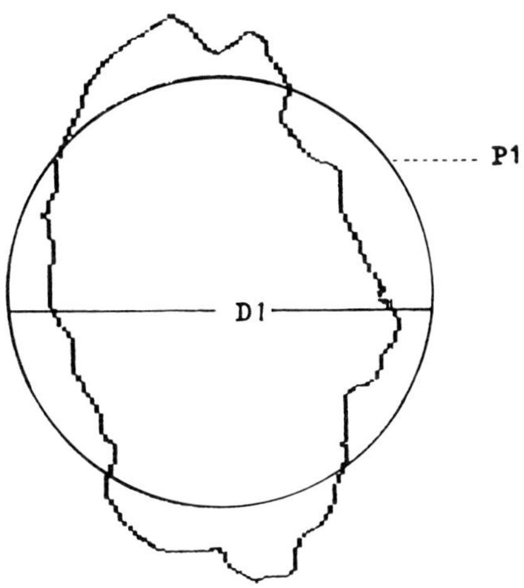

Fig. 10. The diameter of circle equivalent to measured area (the same tubule as shown in Fig. 9)

P1 is the outer perimeter of a given tubule; P2 is the perimeter of the enclosed ring closest to the lumen along the nucleus margin (obtained by tracing the edge of the nucleus); P3 is the inner perimeter of the tubule. A1, A2, and A3 represent the areas enclosed by P1, P2 and P3, respectively.

Calculation of D1, D2 and D3 values, each representing the diameters of a circle equivalent to one of the above areas (A1, A2, and A3), is carried out using the following formulas:

$$A = \pi r^2$$

$$r = \sqrt{\frac{A}{\pi}}$$

$$D1 = 2r1$$
$$D2 = 2r2$$
$$D3 = 2r3$$

P1/D1 represents the irregularity of tubule structure. P2/D2 is the ratio of perimeter obtained by tracing the edge of nuclei nearest to the lumen of the dysplastic tubule to the diameter of its equivalent circle. The nuclei are in the space between P1 and P2 whose width is equal to r1 − r2; the area enclosed by P1 and P3 represents a tubule wall width equal to r1 − r3; N/C should be calculated as:

$$N/C = \frac{r1 - r2}{r1 - r3}$$

This is based on P1, P2, and P3, obtained from normal pyloric and metaplastic tubules in 26 cases, obvious moderate dysplastic tubules in 14 cases, and well differentiated carcinomatous tubules in 14 cases. The standard values of N/C, P1/D1 and P2/D2 are presented in Table 1.

In gastric dysplasia, histological changes are usually to be seen when its tubules are decribed as distorting, "budding", or branching, or showing papillary growth, etc. These changes can be expressed as P1/D1 and P2/D2 values. Because the P2/D2 value is also determined by cellular atypia such as the uniformity and the arrangement of nuclei, P2/D2 expresses not only histological (structural) but also cellular atypia.

These indexes are now also to be found as a designed computer program, and a clinical trial has been carried out [34]. Owing to the fact that

Table 1. Measurement value for grading dysplasia

Index	Normal	Dysplasia					Cancer	
		Mild		Moderate		Severe		
N/C	0.3637	——	0.5306	——	0.6046	——	0.6640	——
P1/D1	3.6037	——	3.6538	——	3.9278	——	4.1050	——
P2/D2	3.8880	——	4.4045	——	4.8685	——	4.9287	——

morphometric indexes are mainly objective, pathologists should benefit greatly and new standards set. It is hoped, also, that there will be further new indexes of this character [30, 37].

Malignant Change in Gastric Dysplasia

Gastric dysplasia has been regarded as precancerous because pathologists have found that some of these lesions are transformed into gastric cancer. The following sections deal with the two ways in which cancerous change in gastric dysplasia may be researched.

Histopathological Judging Criteria

From the relationship of the topographic distribution of the cancerously transformed foci within the dysplastic lesion, there are histological findings enough to verify malignant change in gastric dysplasia. Figure 2 is a case of adenomatous dysplasia of intestinal type, and a cancerously changed focus was detected in the dysplastic lesion. Regardless of architectures or epithelial cells, there were striking differences between the dysplastic and cancerous portions, but sometimes a transitional zone could be found. The author believes that in such a cases a small part of the dysplastic lesion had changed into cancer, thus ruling out the possibility that many foci with different degrees of differentiation had occurred within the same early polypoid cancer. If this possibility is not ruled out, then we can also eliminate the possibility that a concomitant dysplasia occurred near the cancer focus.

In some other cases of early or advanced gastric cancer, dysplastic foci (single or multiple) accompany the cancer focus. Most of the multiple dysplastic foci are distributed near the cancer focus. When we come to consider which of the dysplastic foci seen on the cancer-bearing stomach specimens occurred before the cancer and which occurred after the cancer, it can be said that it was clearly found in our patients, i.e., in 41 cases of early gastric cancer, that 16 (39%) were accompanied by gastric dysplasia, whereas in our 531 cases of advanced gastric cancer, only 25 cases (4.7%) were accompanied by gastric dysplasia. If the dysplasias had occurred after the cancer, more dysplastic foci should have been be seen in the stomach bearing advanced cancer. There were, however, more dysplastic foci around the early gastric cancers than around the advanced one. This phenomenon can only be explained if it is accepted that the gastric cancer occurred on the basis of the dysplastic lesions of the stomach. It can be said, also, that few dysplastic foci were found around a single gastric cancer, i.e., 30/543 cases (5.5%). By contrast, far more dysplastic foci were to be seen around multiple cancers, i.e., 11/26 cases (42.3%). This supports the view that the early foci of some of the cancers, occurred on the basis of the dysplastic lesions [39].

In summarizing cancerous change in dysplastic lesions, the following points should be considered. First, if the cancer focus occurred on the basis of gastric dysplasia, there is reliable evidence to suggest that the dysplastic lesion serves as a greater part of the focus than the cancerous portion. In other words, the smaller the quantity of cancerous tissues, the easier it is to identify that part of the dysplastic lesion which is cancerous. Second, if the dysplasias are the basic lesions of cancerous change, there must be a distinct difference between the dysplasia and the cancer. Eliminating, as far as possible, overlapping or fusion of a separately occurring dysplasia and cancer during the process of enlargement of the two separate foci, it can be said that the two different tissues would usually come into contact with each other but that there would be an obvious borderline; transitional features from dysplasia to cancer are not seen.

According to these two histopathological judging criteria, cancerous changes in our cases of gastric dysplasia were as follows.

In 39 cases of adenomatous dysplasia, two were found with malignant transformation (42). Three and 13 cases of malignant change were detected in 65 cryptal and 53 globoid dysplasias [16, 45], while early or primitive cancerous transformations were detected in five of 48 cases of regenerative dysplasia [45].

Follow-up Studies

Follow-up studies of gastric dysplasia are carried out so that more might be known about the relationship between gastric dysplasia and gastric cancer, i.e., developments and changes within the dysplastic lesions might be observed by gastroscope and mucosal biopsy. This is a rather difficult examination to carry out as many dysplastic lesions are occasionally detected in pathologic sections of mucosal biopsies except for the small number of visible protruded (adenomatous) dysplastic foci. Reexamination of the site where a certain abnormal change had been detected in the gastric mucosa when it had been under gastroscope for the first time, is carried out after a definite period of time, and it is difficult to pinpoint the biopsied site again. For that reason, much care has to be shown during the follow-up study, and a skillful microscopic examination is important.

Several local and international registration units have been detailed to perform this difficult study. One was organized by the International Study Group in Gastric Cancer (ISGGC) during the workshop held at San Miniato, Florence, Italy, in 1982 [19]. Another was organized at the WHO-CC (Tokyo) meeting in 1987 [33].

We had followed up many cases showing varying degrees of gastric dysplasia [43]. Among them, cancerous changes were found to be frequent.

There was one case (during a mass survey in January 1975) in which granular lesions in the antrum and erosions in the gastric notch were detected, and evidence of erosions with repairing processes and disorganized architecture of the mucosa was found histopathologically. Moderate or severe atypia of the mucosa, accompanied by chronic gastritis were diagnosed. During reexamination in November 1976, the microscopic diagnosis was severe chronic gastritis with moderate atypical hyperplasia. Malignancy could not be affirmed but conservative treatment was needed because of the possibility of severe lesions. During further reexamination by mucosal biopsies in January 1977 the poorly differentiated adenocarcinoma was proved. The surgically resected stomach specimen was verified as type IIc early gastric cancer.

Another case was examined gastroscopically in May 1975 and a 1.0 × 1.5 cm round shallow ulcer was found in the anterior wall of the pyloric region, with much mucus covering the central portion of the ulcer. The mucosa of the lesser curvature of the pyloric region was rough. In mucosal biopsy specimen, it was found that the pyloric glands were strikingly disorganized. Their shapes were irregular and some were dilated. The epithelial cells showed marked atypia indicating moderate dysplastic change. In the following year, further mucosal biopsies were carried out and moderate dysplasia was detected, while dysplastic epithelial cells showed marked atypia. A third reexamination in November 1977 revealed more obvious atypia of the gastric tubules and epithelium than that seen before. Necrotic materials were also detected in some tubules. Histopathological diagnosis was severe dysplasia, and malignancy was suspected. Surgical resection was then suggested. On the stomach specimen, a small (1.5 × 1.3 cm) superficial early gastric cancer of type IIa + IIc at the lesser curvature of the pyloric region was seen. Its histopathological feature was well differentiated adenocarcinoma while there was a penetrating spot into the submucosa in the center of the cancer focus, and early metastasis was detected in a drainage lymph node. It can be said of the above-mentioned two cases, that as the sites of repeated mucosal biopsies showed a consistent trend, it was possible to decide histopathologically that the changes seen were the cancerous changes of gastric dysplasias.

Summary

How many gastric dysplasias transform to cancer? Does a dysplastic lesion remain unchanged for a long time in the process of its development, or disappear, or become gastric cancer? And what types or grades of dysplasia can disappear or develop cancerously? Answering these questions is rather difficult, notwithstanding the many reports of follow-up studies in the literature. Nagayo's latest retrospective histological studies on biopsies for gastric lesions affirmed that in most of his 41 studied cases cancerous changes were detected during follow-up at the location of the original lesions; reexamination of the biopsied specimens taken at the first examination revealed that in 33 (80.5%) no precancerous atypical changes appeared to have occurred [23]. This is a very interesting report which deserves consideration. In addition, further studies of precancerous changes of the gastric mucosa are necessary.

References

1. Borchard P, Mitteistaedt A, Stux G (1979) Dysplasien im Resektionsmagen und Klassifikationsprobleme verschiedener Dysplasieformen. Verh Dtsch Ges Pathol 63:250–257
2. Bordi C, de Vita O (1984) Pathologia delle precancerosi gastriche e colorektali estratio. Argom Oncol 5:323–331
3. Cuello C, Correa P, Zarama G, Lopez J, Murrar J, Gordillo G (1979) Histopathology of gastric dysplasia. Am J Surg Pathol 3:491–500
4. Fukuji S, Kaiyama M, Nozotsuki K (1975) Endoscopic diagnosis of IIa-subtype borderline lesion of the stomach (in Japanese). Stomach Intest 10:1487–1493
5. Grundman E, Schlake W (1979) Histology of possible precancerous stages in stomach. In: Herfarth C, Schlag P (eds) Gastric cancer. Springer, Berlin Heidelberg New York, pp 72–82
6. Hirota T, Itabashi M, Takizawa C, Kim B (1987) Clinicopathological characteristics of gastric adenoma and its significance as a precancerous lesion (in Japanese). Stomach Intest 22:657–664
7. Japanese Research Society for Gastric Cancer (1985) The general rules for the gastric cancer study, 11th edn. Kanabara, Tokyo, pp 78–100
8. Jarvis L, Whitehead K (1985) Morphometric analysis of gastric dysplasia. J Pathol 147:133–138
9. Jass JR (1980) Role of intestinal metaplasia in the histogenesis of gastric carcinoma. J Clin Pathol 33:801–810
10. Jass JR (1988) Classification of gastric dysplasia. Histopathology 7:181–193
11. Kikuchi M, Nakamura K, Akabane H, Shibuya S (1984) Objectification of histologic diagnosis on protruded lesion of atypical epithelium and differentiated carcinoma of stomach: numerical value of structural atypism by morphometric analysis (Engl summary). Stomach Intest 19:1117–1125
12. Li JY, Ho L, Xie YQ, He JS, Jin BQ (1989) Cystic dilatation of the dysplastic gland in gastric mucosa and its relation with gastric cancer (in Chinese). Chinese J Dig 9:230–231
13. Liu SQ, Zhang YC (1987) A newly recognized precancerous lesion of the stomach (Engl abstr). J China Med Univ 16:321–325
14. Liu SQ, Zhang YC (1988) The histopathological classification of globoid dysplasia and its relationship with signet ring cell carcinoma (Engl abstr). J China Med Univ 17:1–6
15. Liu SQ, Zhang YC (1988) The cellular histochemical and immunohistochemical studies on the globoid dysplasia of the human gastric epithelium (Engl abstr). J China Med Univ 17:92–102
16. Liu SQ, Zhang YC (1989) Histopathologic features of globoid dysplasia of the human gastric epithelium (Engl abstr). Chung Hua Chung Liu Tsa Chin 11:37–40
17. Liu SQ, Zhang YC (1989) Characteristics of mucins and CEA in globoid dysplastic cells of human stomach and its relationship with signet ring cell carcinoma (Engl abstr). Zhonghua Zhongliu Zazhi (Chin J Oncol) 11:176–179

18. Ming SC (1984) Precursors of gastric cancer. Praeger, New York
19. Ming SC, Bajtai A, Correa P, Elster K, Jarvi OH, Munoz N, Nagayo T, Stemmerman GN (1984) Gastric dysplasia. Significance and pathologic criteria. Cancer 54: 1794–1800
20. Morson BC, Sobin LH, Grundmann E, Johansen A, Nagayo T, Serck-Hanssen A (1980) Precancerous conditions and epithelial dysplasia in the stomach. J Clin Pathol 33:711–721
21. Nagayo T (1982) Gastric mucosal dysplasia and precancerous lesion (in Japanese). In: Kusama S, Wada T, Miye M (eds) Surgery, vol 28. Kanabara, Tokyo
22. Nagayo T (1986) Histogenesis and precursors of human gastric cancer. Springer, Berlin Heidelberg New York, pp 126–140
23. Nagayo T, Suzuki R, Sato T, Suchi T (1987) Retrospective histological studies on biopsied gastric lesions of patients in whom cancer was diagnosed at follow-up examination. Gann 78:997–1005
24. Nakamura K (1982) Structure of the gastric cancer, 1st edn (in Japanese). Igaku-Shoin, Tokyo
25. Nakamura K, Sugano H, Takagi K, Fuchigami A (1966) Histopathological study or early carcinoma of the stomach. Criteria for diagnosis of atypical epithelium. Gann 57:613–620
26. Nakamura K, Sakaguchi H, Enjoji M (1988) Depressed adenoma of the stomach. Cancer 62:2197–2202
27. Oehler W (1979) Biological significance of dysplasia of the epithelium and of atrophic gastritis. In: Herfarth CH, Schlag P (eds) Gastric cancer. Springer, Berlin Heidelberg New York, pp 91–104
28. Sano L (1975) Benign and malignant borderline lesions of the stomach (in Japanese). Stomach Intest 10:1433–1435
29. Sugano H (1972) The pathological morphology of the borderline lesion in digestive tract: atypical epithelium of the stomach (in Japanese). Gan No Rinsho 18:834–842
30. Wang RN, Zhao ML, Su, BH, Ziao SD, Jiang SJ (1988) A model assessment of gastric precancerous lesions by morphometric analysis. Chin Med J [Engl] 101: 403–409
31. Watanabe H (1978) Argentaffin cells in adenoma of the stomach. Cancer 30: 1267–1274
32. World Health Organization (1972) Report of a WHO meeting on the histological definition of precancerous lesions. WHO, Geneva
33. World Health Organization (1987) Establishment of international registration system for gastric dysplasia. WHO CC News Lett 18
34. Wu YQ, Yen RF, Zhang YC (1988) Computer diagnosis of gastric dysplasia and program design (Engl abstr). Zhonghua Zhongliu Zazhi (Chin J Oncol) 10:24–26
35. Xiao SD, Jiang SJ, Wang RN, Hu YB, Liu WZ, Tang XM (1986) N-ethyl-N′-nitro-N-nitrosoguanidine induced gastric carcinoma in wolf-dogs – useful model for tracing gastric malignancy transformation. Chin Med J [Engl] 99:903–907
36. Yen RF, Zhang YC, Wu YQ (1987) Morphological measurement for diagnosis of gastric dysplasia (Engl abstr). Zhonghua Zhongliu Zazhi (Chin J Oncol) 9:401–404
37. Yen RF, Zhang YC, Wu YQ (1989) Morphometric indexes and computerized diagnosis of gastric dysplasia. Proc CAMS and PUMC 4:43–47
38. Zhang YC (1983) Epithelial dysplasia of the stomach and its relationship with gastric cancer. 6th Asia Pacific Cancer Conference, Sendi
39. Zhang YC (1984) Epithelial dysplasia of the stomach and its relationship with gastric cancer. In: Ming SC (ed) Precursors of gastric cancer. Praeger, New York, pp 41–52
40. Zhang YC (1988) Gastric dysplasia. In: Zhang YC (ed) Pathology of the stomach and gastric mucosal biopsy (in Chinese). Liaoning, Shenyang pp 56–74
41. Zhang YC (1989) Pathology of the start point of malignant change from gastric dysplasia (Engl abstr). J Chin Med Univ 18:337–341
42. Zhang YC (1990) Malignant change detected in regenerative type of gastric dysplasia. 79th Meeting of the Japanese Pathologic Association, Fukuoka

43. Zhang YC, Bai XZ, Zhang WF (1979) Histopathologic study of atypical epithelial proliferation of the gastric mucosa and its follow-up study (Engl abstr). Zhonghua Zhongliu Zazhi (Chin J Oncol) 1:23–28
44. Zhang YC, Sun ZX, Lin HZ, Zhang WF, Bai XW, Aoki K, Kawai K, Sasaki R, Tsychihashi Y, Ito Y, Watanabe N (1987) Spectrum of gastric diseases in North China. In: Wada T, Aoki K, Yachi A (eds) Current status of cancer research in Asia, the Middle East and other countries. UICC-JCA joint conference. University of Nagoya Press, Nagoya, pp 41–49
45. Zhang YC, Zhang PF, Wang MX, Liu SQ (1988) Histopathologic types of gastric dysplasia. Chin J Cancer Res 1:47–52
46. Zhao ML, Wang RN, Deng YL, Yao JS, Xiao SD, Jiang SJ, Ju HG, Chen DH, Li ZP (1985) A morphometric analysis of gastric precancerous lesions. Quantitative diagnosis of structural atypism in gastric mucosal biopsies. Chin J Dig 5:205–206

7 Precancerous Changes of the Stomach Observed in Surgical Specimens and Biopsy Materials

T. Nagayo

Introduction

The term "precursor" includes two different concepts – precancerous disease or condition and precancerous change or lesion. "Precancerous condition" is a clinical term meaning, from statistical viewpoints that the condition has a higher risk of cancerization than nondiseased stomach, "Precancerous lesion", on the other hand, is a histological term implying that the premalignant nature of the lesion can only be known by histological examination. Thus, the two terms are by no means synonymous, but it is also true that all precancerous lesions of the stomach are found in gastric diseases that can be diagnosed clinically as precancerous conditions (Fig. 1).

Precancerous Diseases of the Stomach

Several types of precancerous diseases of the stomach, e.g., gastric polyp, chronic peptic ulcer, chronic atrophic gastritis, gastric remnant, and pernicious anemia, will be described before the histological nature of precancerous lesions are described.

Gastric Polyp

Regardless of size, site and shape, gastric polyps are defined macroscopically as focal proliferation of gastric mucosa showing hemispheric, pedunculated or sessile forms and having, in some cases, a smooth or lobulated surface, and in others a granular or strawberry-like appearance. The number and size of the polyps also vary from a single, large polyp to multiple, tiny ones but they are mostly unifocal and less than 2 cm in diameter. The site of the polyp is random, there being no preferential site. Tiny or small polyps without any clinical symptoms are not uncommon in the stomach.

Aichi Cancer Center, Nagoya, Japan

Ying-Chan Zhang/Keiichi Kawai (Eds.)
Precancerous Conditions and Lesions of the Stomach

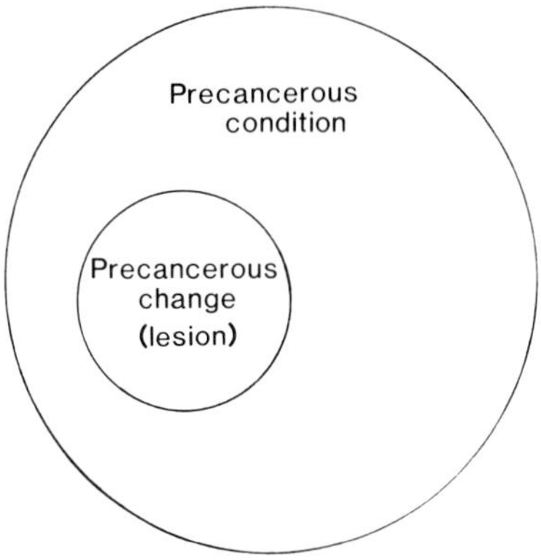

Fig. 1. Relation between precancerous condition and precancerous change

Table 1. Characteristics of hyperplastic polyps

Balanced proliferation of constituents of gastric mucosa
1. Elongation and branching of foveolar tissue
2. Proliferation of pyloric or fundic glands
3. Proliferation of stromal connective tissue
4. Fountain-like contour of muscularis mucosae
Other changes often present
a. Edema of the stroma
b. Erosion of mucosal surface
c. Cystic dilatation of the glands
d. Increase of mucus production

When the real frequency of malignant transformation of epithelial gastric polyps is sought, the method of detection should not be based on surgically resected stomachs but on endoscopically detectable polyps, because of the highly restricted surgical resectability of the polyps. For this reason, biopsy specimens taken from consecutively followed-up cases of gastric polyps by the aid of endoscope were used for the examination.

On the basis of their histological natures, the biopsied gastric polyps were classified into two main types: (a) hyperplastic, and (b) adenomatous. The characteristics of both types are summarized in Tables 1, 2.

The 198 consecutive cases of gastric polyp detected and biopsied during the 8 years from 1966 to 1974 were serially examined. Among them, 175 cases (87.6%) were diagnosed histologically as hyperplastic polyp, while 13 cases (6.6%) were diagnosed as adenomatous polyp. In another ten cases, classification could not be made owing to the poor quality of the materials. Malignant changes were seen in only one case of hyperplastic polyp, which was exceptionally large (more than 2 cm in diameter) and in nine cases of adenomatous polyp. From these results, the rate of coexistence of malignancy in the gastric polyps was calculated as 0.6% in the hyperplastic polyps and 69.2% in the adenomatous polyps (Table 3).

Table 2. Characteristics of adenomatous polyps

Adenomatous proliferation composed solely of foveolar tissue
1. Irregular growth of metaplastic foveolar tissue
2. Atrophy of pyloric or fundic glands
3. Compression of stroma by the epithelial growth
4. Fountain like contour of muscularis mucosae

Other changes often present
a. Decrease in number of goblet cells
b. Cystic dilatation of tubules or glands
c. Appearance of atypical epithelia
d. Appearance of cancerous epithelia

Table 3. Frequencies of hyperplastic and adenomatous polyps and rate of association with cancer as detected by histological examination of biopsies

Diagnosis	Cases	
	No.	%
Hyperplastic polyp (HP)	174	87.8
Adenomatous polyp (AP)	4	2.0
Unclassified	10	5.1
Cancer in polyp	10 < 1 (HP), 9 (AP)	5.1
Total	198	100.0

Hyperplastic polyp $\frac{1}{174+1} \times 100 = 0.6\%$

Adenomatous polyp $\frac{9}{4+9} \times 100 = 69.2\%$

$$\frac{10}{198} \times 100 = 5.1\%$$

It can therefore be said that most gastric polyps diagnosed by means of X-ray and/or endoscopy are hyperplastic in nature, and this type of polyp rarely undergoes malignant transformation, unless it is more than 2 cm in diameter. Gastric polyp of the adenomatous type is far more likely to become malignant, as are cases of colorectal polyps.

Chronic Gastric Ulcer

Peptic ulcer is one of the commonest diseases of the stomach. The site, size, shape, depth, and, of course, stage of the ulcer are various. From the

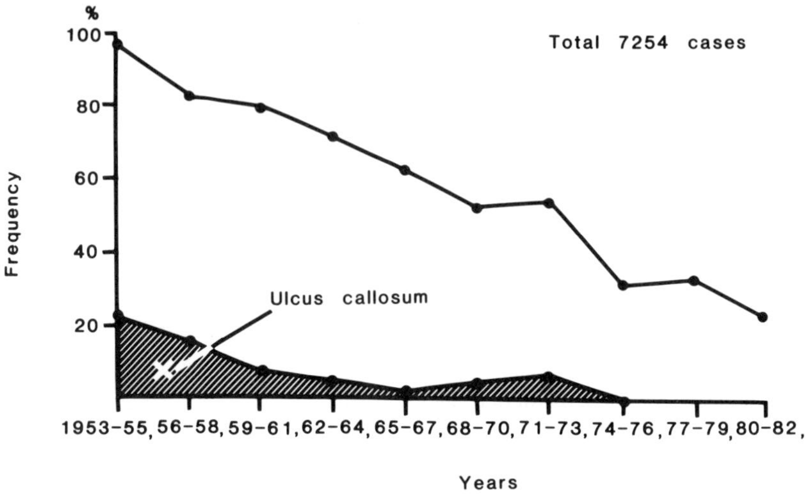

Fig. 2. Annual change in frequency of chronic gastric ulcer among total gastric ulcers resected

aspect of histogenesis of gastric cancer, however, only chronic type ulcers are concerned and nonchronic ones bear almost no relation to malignant transformation.

Chronic peptic ulcer is characterized by the presence of an open, deep and hard ulcer accompanied by shortening of the lesser curvature and convergency of the mucosal folds toward the center of the ulcer due to intensive fibrosis at the base of the ulcer. Even barium-filled X-ray examinations are able to detect such a lesions without too much difficulty, owing to the ulcer's characteristic deformity and presence of niche.

In about 1955, such chronic peptic ulcers were commonest in resected stomachs. Among these ulcers, cases showing cancerous change in the mucosa around the ulcer were not infrequent, and many of them fulfilled the histological criteria of "Ulcer-cancer" proposed by Hauser. On the basis of these results, the author came to the conclusion that cancerization can often occur in the mucosa around chronic gastric ulcer.

Since then, however, the incidence of gastric cancer seemingly preceded by chronic ulcer has decreased year by year until, in recent years, such cases have seldom been observed. The main reason for this dramatic decline must be the marked decrease in the number of chronic peptic ulcers (Fig. 2).

During more than 30 years of histological examinations of resected stomachs, the average frequency of early gastric cancer with histological evidence of the ulcer-cancer sequence among the total gastric ulcers resected has been calculated as 1.4% (96/7023).

Chronic Atrophic Gastritis and Intestinal Metaplasia

From studies of histogenesis, the frequency of early gastric cancer (EGC) showing histological evidence of polyp-cancer or ulcer-cancer sequences among a total of 1109 EGC cases examined was calculated at <15%, as expressed by a dark, oblique line in Fig. 3.

These results definitively confirm the importance of the role of a flat mucosa – atrophic or hypertrophic – in possible precancerous conditions of the stomach. It has already been pointed out by many clinical investigators that most patients suffering from long-standing stomach disorders have some degree of hypoacidity or sometimes achlorhydria without any focal mucosal lesions, and that this is generally more frequent in elderly than young people. From the viewpoint of clinical pathology, hypoacidity results from atrophy of acid-secreting parietal cells of the fundic gland, while atrophy of gastrin- and mucin-secreting pyloric glands is also involved. The atrophic changes of the mucosa are quite often observed in the stomach affected by EGC. For these reasons, chronic atrophic gastritis has been cited as one of the most important precursors of gastric cancer.

When atrophy of the gastric glands, especially in pyloric gland areas, becomes diffuse and intensive, foveolar epithelia comprising the upper layer of the mucosa always transforms into the metaplastic intestinal type, characterized by tall, columnar epithelia with a brush border, goblet cells and cells with Paneth's granules. The metaplastic changes usually appear first in the atrophic mucosa of the antrum or of the angulus along the lesser curvature, and then extend gradually to the surrounding mucosa. Intestinal metaplasia of gastric mucosa is, therefore, a histological marker for identifying the grade of the mucosal atrophy.

Histological studies on EGC have confirmed that intestinal metaplasia of gastric mucosa is closely correlated with the development of gastric cancer, especially that of intestinal-type histology. However, owing to the limitations of the study, a causal relationship between the two changes is still

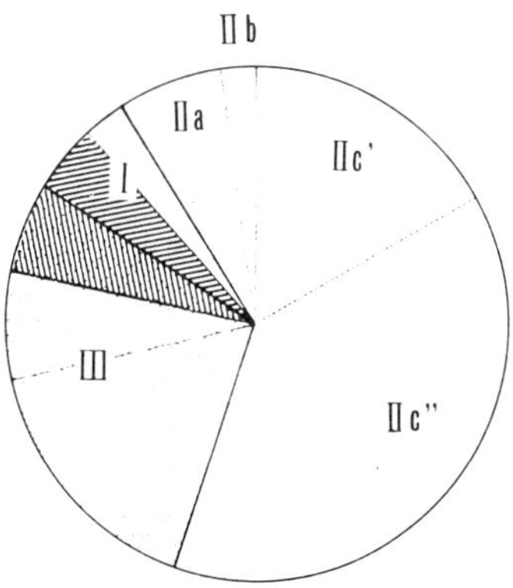

Fig. 3. Relative frequency of the various stages of gastric cancer

Table 4. Differences of complete and incomplete type of intestinal metaplasia in stomach

Marker	Intestinal metaplasia		Small intestine	Large intestine
	Complete type	Incomplete type		
Cell				
Goblet cell	+	+	+	+
Paneth cell	+	−	+	−
Mucus				
HID	−	+	−	+
Enzyme				
Succurase	+	+	+	−
Treharase	+	−	+	−
LAP	+	+	+	−
AIP	+	−	+	−

not clear. As shown in Table 4, intestinal metaplasia of gastric mucosa can be classified into two types – complete and incomplete – and the results of recent investigations suggest that the incomplete type metaplasia with sulfomucin is more likely to promote the development of gastric cancer (Table 4).

At all events, a long-standing condition progressing towards the atrophy of gastric glands seems a necessary factor for the development of gastric cancer, and these changes can be known by endoscopic examination with biopsy.

Pernicious Anemia

The characteristic feature of pernicious anemia is hypoproteinemia and atrophy of the mucosa of the corpus and/or fundus, leaving the mucosa of the antrum intact, and there are geographic differences in its occurrence. Histologically, atrophy of the mucosa of corpus is due to marked atrophy of the fundic glands, composed of chief cells, parietal cells and mucous neck cells, responsible for the secretion of acidic gastric juice. The clinical diagnosis, therefore, is based chiefly on roentgenologic-, endoscopic- and blood examinations. Intestinal metaplasia confined to the musoca of corpus and/or fundus is generally quite rare in the ordinary gastric mucosa but it is not uncommon in pernicious anemia.

Many papers stress that the risk of developing gastric cancer is much higher in patients suffering from pernicious anemia than in the general population. The cancerous lesions derived from this disease also have a predilection for the mucosa of the corpus and/or fundus. On the basis of findings reported, it is supposed that histogenesis of gastric cancer derived from pernicious anemia is not essentially different from that of cancer derived from the ordinary type of chronic atrophic gastritis. From the viewpoints of pathogenesis and etiology, however, the disease is characterized by genetic background, and an autoimmune nature of the disease is suspected by some investigators.

Gastric Remnant

A gastric remnant is the part of the stomach remaining after partial gastrectomy. In gastric remnants, such changes as stomal ulcer, polypoid mucosal protrusion, or cancer can occur many years after the gastrectomy, and these changes are most often found in the gastric mucosa adjacent to gastroduodenal or gastrojejunal anastomoses. Cancer that has developed in a gastric remnant is generally called "stump carcinoma' but from the standpoint of histogenesis, it would be better if this term was confined to cancer developing in the gastric remnant after partial resection of nonmalignant lesions (most of which are peptic ulcers) for eliminating the possibility of recurrence of cancer. In fact, most investigators reporting on this subject have defined stump caricinoma in this way. Furthermore, there is general agreement that in order to eliminate the possibility that the cancer already existed in the upper half of the stomach at the time of surgical operation and was overlooked, the interval between gastrectomy and the detection of cancer in the gastric remnants must be over 5 years. Since it is not unusual for stump carcinoma to develop more than 15 years after gastrectomy, gastric remnant has been cited as a possible precancerous condition of the stomach [1].

However, there are still differences of opinion as to whether gastric remnants carry a higher risk than nonresected stomachs. Most investigators support the view that gastric remnants hold the greater risk. The frequency of stump carcinoma depends on the interval between surgical resection and the date of detection. For this reason, it is necessary to carry out an age-adjusted statistical comparison 15, 20, 25, and 30 years after the partial gastrectomy.

Most papers, including our own, point out that the frequency of stump carcinoma is higher following the Billroth II resection procedure than after the Billroth I, and the cancers were most often seen in the gastric mucosa adjacent to the anastomosis. It is also mentioned by almost all authors that the average interval between gastrectomy and detection of cancer in the gastric remnants is more than 15 years.

These results have brought about general acceptance of the opinion that long-standing refluxed bile flow play an essential role in the development of cancer, especially at the site of anastomoses.

Similar results were obtained from our own examination. There were 27 cancerous lesions in the 25 patients, the primary diseases being gastric ulcer in 13, duodenal ulcer in 11, and 'other' in one. Among them, eight lesions

Table 5. Methods of initial surgery and sites of cancer in stomach remnant

Site of cancer / Method of surgery	Anastomosis	Cardia	Other	Total number of lesions
Billroth II (17 cases)	12	1	6	19
Billroth I (8 cases)	0	5	3	8
Total	12	6	9	27

were found in the stomachs after Billroth I resection procedure, while the other 19 lesions were in the stomachs after the Billroth II procedure. Carinoma at the site of anastomosis accounted for 12 cases (63.2%) in the Billroth II stomachs, but none in the Billroth I stomachs [4] (Table 5).

More than 50% of the cancers were sited in the gastric mucosa adjacent to the anastomosis, and they did not appear until more than 15 years after surgery. Protruding lesions with the histology of poorly differentiated, medullary adenocarcinomas were relatively frequent. Background lesion, which is characteristic of this disease, will be explained in the next section of this chapter.

We succeeded in inducing cancerous lesions similar in nature to stump carcinoma in a large proportion of rats (around 45%) by the application of a specifically designed surgical procedure, which forced duodenal contents to regurgitate into the partially resected stomachs without any use of a known chemical carcinogen [2].

Ménétrier's Disease and Aberrant Pancreas

Gastric cancer can occur on the basis of Ménétrier's disease. The characteristic features of this disease are giant hypertrophy of the mucosal folds, similar in appearance to gyri of the brain, in an area of the corpus and fundus, with hypoproteinemia. Histologically, remarkable proliferation of all the fundic glands without prominent structural abnormality is a characteristic feature of Ménétrier's disease. A few cases of malignant transformation of this disease on the surface of the hypertrophic mucosa have been reported and we also experienced such a case.

Aberrant pancreas is by no means uncommon in the stomach, showing the macroscopical appearance of a focal submucosal tumor, but cases showing histological evidence of malignant transformation of these aberrant pancreatic tissues – mostly ductules – are exceptionally rare.

Precancerous Lesions of the Stomach

As stressed in the introduction, precancerous lesions should be defined as lesions which are already in the course of cancerization but still do not fulfill the histological criteria of malignancy. The lesion is recognizable only by histological examination. We are, therefore, describing precancerous change, in the strict sense of these words.

In approaching this study, two methods are available, one a histological examination of surgically resected stomachs and the other follow-up of suspected precancerous lesions histologically with the aid of endocopic biopsy.

In the first method, the lesion is infrequently composed of precancerous change alone, owing to its limited resectability. It is, however, by no means rare to detect precancerous tissue changes within or adjacent to the obvious lesion of adenocarcinoma by scrutinized histological examination of the lesions, and also precancerous lesions quite close to the very site at which carcinoma in situ began to develop.

The second method is a more direct way of detecting histological and chronological change from precancer to cancer, even though there are many limited conditions and painstaking effort is required.

When carring out histological diagnosis of precancerous lesions, it is necessary to be well acquainted with the term "dysplasia" [5, 8]. As proposed by the WHO Committee on Histological Criteria of Precancerous Changes of the Stomach [6], based on the grades of (a) cellular atypia, (b) abnormal differentiation, and (c) disorganized mucosal architecture, dysplasia can be classified into three groups – mild, moderate and severe [8, 9, 10, 11] (Table 6).

Mild dysplasia is seen in several kinds of histological changes, ranging from regenerative but maturation-arrested epithelia following deep erosion to hyperplastic lesion with slight structural derangement. In general, the lesion that can be diagnosed as showing mild dysplasia displays no histological changes that are likely to become malignant, and, because of the superficial nature of the changes, some of them can regress to the normal state. This reversal of dysplasia is seen in both elevated and depressed mucosae, but the histological features suggest that reversibility to non-dysplastic mucosae is more frequent in the latter.

The borderline lesion with broad-based and flat mucosal elevation is a typical example of *moderate dysplasia* [7]. Prominent disorganized mucosal architecture, especially with many large glandular cysts, decreased numbers of goblet cells in the metaplastic tubules, and an increase of mitotic cells in the atypically proliferated epithelia, means irreversibility of the lesions. The possibility that the lesion will progress to a severe grade of dysplasia or transform directly into carcinoma cannot be ruled out, but in the cases of broad-based mucosal elevations, the condition of the atypically proliferative epithelia is mostly stationary.

Table 6. Comparison of different grading systems for gastric dysplasia

Nagayo (1971)	No atypia	Slight atypia	Borderline	Probable cancer	Cancer
Grundman (1979)	Inflammatory	Mild dysplasia	Moderate dysplasia	Severe dysplasia	
Oehlert (1979)		Grade I	Grade II	Grade III	
Ming (1979)	Grade 1	Grade 2	Grade 3	Grade 4	
Cuello (1979)	Hyperplastic mild	Dysplasia severe	Adenomatous mild	Dysplasia severe	
Morson (1980)	Inflammatory regenerative	Mild dysplasia	Moderate dysplasia	Severe dysplasia	
ISGGC[a] (1982)	——— Hyperplasia ———		——— Dysplasia ———		
	simple	atypical		Possible carcinoma	

[a] International Study Group of Gastric Cancer

In contrast to mild and moderate dysplasia, *severe dysplasia* is very close to the state of carcinoma in situ or adenocarcinoma without invasive growth. Indeed, owing to the severe nature of the epithelial and structural changes, it is often difficult to discriminate clearly between the two changes.

Examinations of the Surgically Resected Stomachs

Since the grade of cellular atypia, abnormal differentiation, and disorganization of the mucosal architecture are parallel in most cases, the diagnosis of severe dysplasia is made on the basis of the mucosal changes as a whole, but there are some cases in which the grade of cellular atypia is relatively slight compared with the degree of structural abnormality or vice versa. Nevertheless, it can be said that the essential change in severe dysplasia lies in cellular atypia and not in structure. Differences in the findings between intramucosal cancer and severe dysplasia of the stomach are summarized in Table 7.

It is important to note that in resected stomachs, changes of severe dysplasia are found most frequently in or adjacent to the cancerized mucosa, especially in its early stages, and these changes, being microscopic, have been found even more frequently when scrutinized histologic examinations have been carried out. Owing to several difficulties involved, the frequency of these cases is not known but the raw data show that there are more than 300 cases (ca. 10% among total gastric cancers resected). There were 115 cases of isolated dysplastic lesions, these being apart from the main lesions of cancer or ulcer, mostly the former. Owing to indications of resectability, the lesions with dysplastic changes alone accounted for 40 cases and most of these showed broad-based mucosal elevations with flat surface (Table 8).

Table 7. Differences between the histology of intramucosal cancer from that of severe dysplasia

1. Pleomorphy and loss of polarity of the nuclei are noted
2. Nucleo-cytoplasmic ratio is more markedly increased
3. Loss of cellular differentiation is prominent
4. Abnormal course of the glandular tubules is visible
5. Invasive growth of epithelia into the surrounding stroma
6. Small clusters of glands detaching from neck zone may be seen in nonmetaplastic but atrophic mucosa
7. Epithelium-stroma relationship is disturbed
8. Surface of the affected mucosa loses smoothness and abnormal mitoses may be seen on the surface
9. Whole layers of the mucosa are often occupied by neoplastic tissues
10. Border of the lesion to the surrounding mucosa is serrated to varying degrees

Table 8. Materials used in this study: specimens taken from 16606 stomachs resected during the period 1953–1979

Dysplastic lesions	
— in or adjacent to cancer	Many
— Separate from cancer or ulcer	115 cases
— Alone	40 cases
— Elevated type	31 cases
— Hollowed type (focal atrophy or erosion)	9 cases

Histological evidence indicating malignant transformation of dysplastic lesion can be obtained in several lesions, especially elevated ones (Figs. 4, 5), but this evidence is most frequently found in the case of stomach remnants. The gastric mucosa adjacent to gastrojejunal or gastroduodenal anastomosis often shows elevated lesions with the histology of moderate to severe grade dysplasia, and, in part of the lesion, cancerous changes can be detected (Fig. 6).

The elevated lesions are basically composed of elongated foveolar tubules accompanied by hyperplasia and heterotopic downgrowth of the pseudopyloric glands. The elongated tubules are often twisted or irregularly branched, and glandular cysts are almost always visible in the hyperplastic mucosa. There may or may not be inflammatory cell infiltration in the stroma, together with hyperemia. Intestinal metaplasias are seldom seen in the elevated lesions, and cellular atypia of the tubules and glands is less prominent, in contrast to the high grade of disorganized mucosal architecture. When cancerous changes – mostly of a non-intestinal-type histology – are partly visible in these dysplastic lesions, it is possible to diagnose the lesions as cancer preceded by dysplasia. The author has experienced three cases of such lesions.

It is certain from histological examination of surgically resected stomachs that severe dysplasia is a typical example of a precancerous lesion but from

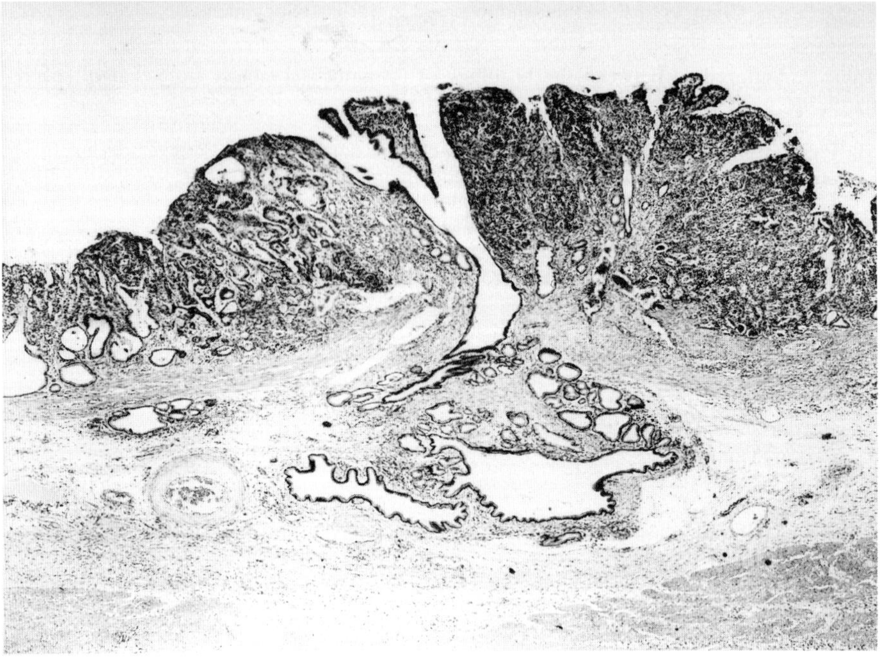

Fig. 4. In the marginal elevated lesion, heterotopic down-growth of the tubules and glands with irregular shaped glandular cysts are visible. In both sides of the aberrant tissue, moderately differentiated (*left side*) and poorly differentiated (*right side*) adenocarcinomas are also visible

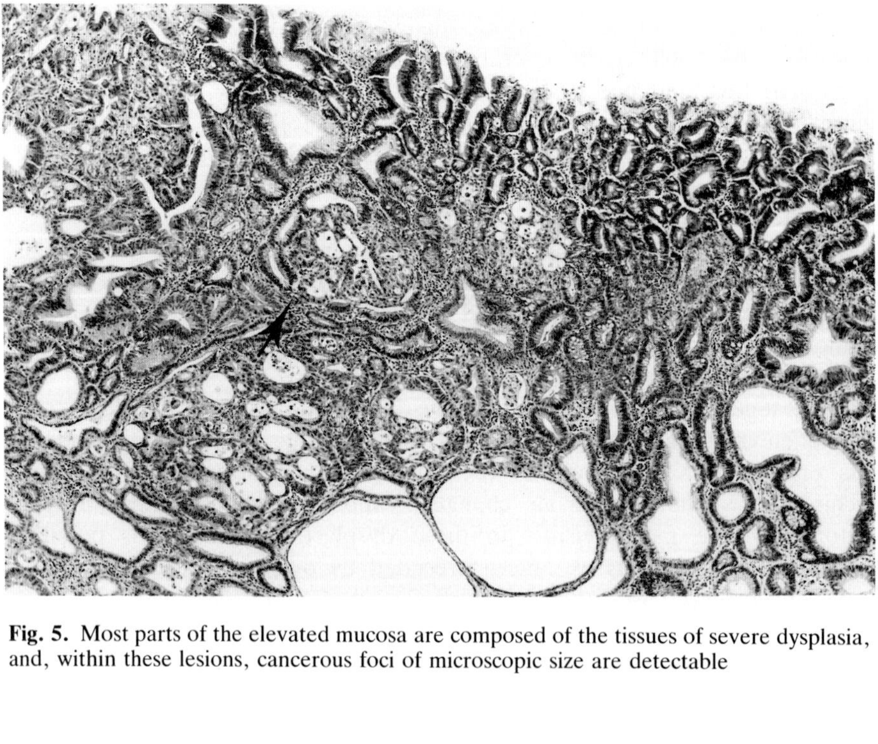

Fig. 5. Most parts of the elevated mucosa are composed of the tissues of severe dysplasia, and, within these lesions, cancerous foci of microscopic size are detectable

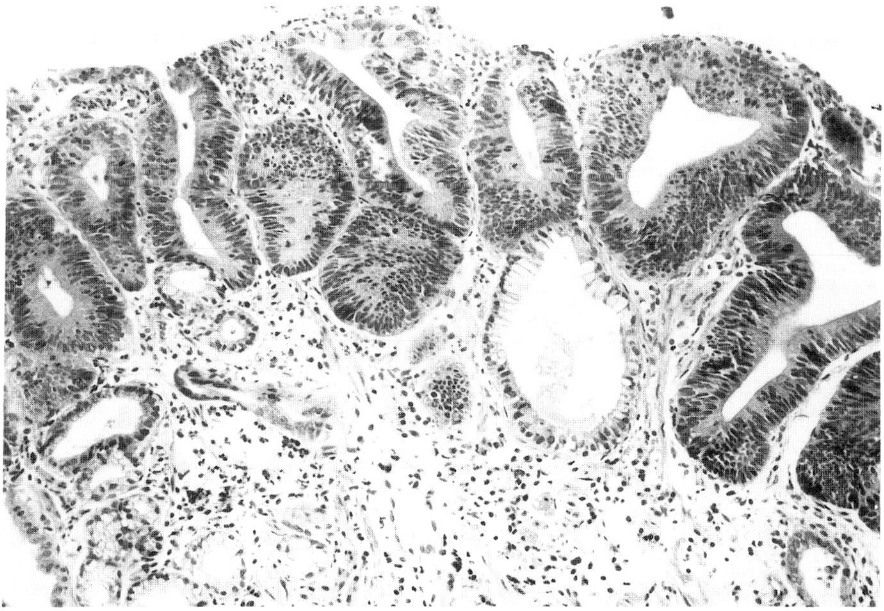

Fig. 6. Biopsied specimens taken from the elevated lesion of the antrum showed the change from moderate to severe dysplasia on its surface. Six years later, the lesion became malignant

this kind of study alone, it is impossible to know the frequency, histology and chronology of malignant transformation of precancerous lesions.

Retrospective Follow-up Examination of the Biopsied Gastric Lesions

In order to study the problem of precancerous changes of the stomach from a clinical viewpoint, retrospective, follow-up, histological examinations of the biopsied specimens taken from the suspected lesions are indispensible. Frequency, nature, and chronology of the putative precancerous lesions can be approached only by this method. For this purpose, the examinations detailed below were carried out [12].

Biopsy specimens taken from gastric mucosae under direct endoscopic observation between 1971 and 1985 in the Aichi Cancer Center Hospital, Nagoya, Japan, were serially reexamined. During this period, 17 429 gastric biopsies were performed and, in 14 779 cases, histological examinations of the biopsied materials were also carried out. Among this vast number of cases, those which had been diagnosed at the first biopsy as benign or non-

Table 9. Frequencies of patients whom cancer was detected in follow-up examinations among patients undergoing endoscopic examinations

Endoscopic diagnosis at first examination	Patients subjected to endoscopic examination twice or more (n)	Patients in whom cancer was detected at reexamination or follow-up	
		(n)	(%)
Open ulcer	521	11	2.1
Ulcer scar	785	13	1.7
Polypoid protrusion	683	6	0.9
Broad-based elevation	239	7	2.9
Erosion, gastritis, etc.	227	4	1.8
Total	2455	41	1.7
Benign lesion	8739	41	0.5

malignant, but in which cancerous changes had been detected in the biopsied specimens during follow-up examinations, were selected.

In these selected cases, the site of the biopsies and the nature of the lesions were carefully examined on the basis of endoscopic records, and the cases were classified into the following three groups:

1. Those in which histological diagnosis of cancer was made by reexamination within 1 year after the first endoscopic examination: 120 cases (most of them diagnosed endoscopically as suspected cancer)
2. Those in which cancerous lesions were detected by endoscopy and biopsy in the mucosa at locations different from the target lesion during the follow-up observations: 34 cases
3. Those in which cancerous changes were detected by endoscopy and biopsy in the target lesion during follow-up observations: 41 cases

For the purpose of the study reported here, only the cases in group 3 were chosen for detailed retrospective histological examinations.

The 41 cases in group 3 amounted to 1.7% of the cases (a total of 2455) that received double, triple or multiple endoscopic examinations with negative results in the biopsies. Benign cases without repeated endoscopic examination amounted to 6284, and, when these cases were added to the denominator, the percentage fell to 0.5% (Table 9).

Macroscopically, the lesions seen at the first endoscopic examination were, in order of frequency, broad-based mucosal elevation, open ulcer, and sessile or pedunculated polyp (Table 9).

Average time intervals between the first and last endoscopic examinations of each type of lesion showed no great difference, but there was a longer interval between these examinations in lesions diagnosed at first

Table 10. Intervals between first examination with endoscopy and biopsy and detection of cancer at follow-up

Endoscopic diagnosis at first examination	Patients in whom cancer was detected during follow-up (*n*)	Period after first examination	
		Average interval (mo)	Range (mo)
Open ulcer	11	38.9	17–84
Ulcer scar	13	57.2	21–150
Polypoid protrusion	6	51.0	26–100
Broad-based elevation	7	48.3	36–64
Erosion, gastritis, etc.	4	66.8	20–133

as erosion or gastritis than between the others (66.8 months, more than 5 years), and the longest interval (150 months, more than 12 years) was seen in the case of ulcer scar (Table 10).

From retrospective examinations of the histologic changes of the group 3 biopsy specimens, it was noticed that the lesions could be further classified into the following three subgroups:

a) Lesions which had shown some diseased conditions in the previous endoscopic examinations, but in which no prominent dysplastic changes were visible in the biopsied specimens.
b) Those displaying a moderate to severe grade of cellular and/or structural atypia suggesting that the precancerous nature of the lesion was observed in the previous histological examinations of the biopsied specimens (Fig. 6).
c) Lesions in which cancerous change, microscopic in size, was found in part of each biopsied specimen on retrospective reexamination (Fig. 7).

Thirty-three cases (80.5%) were classified into subgroup a, six cases (14.6%) into b, and two cases (4.9%) into c. When the cases were limited to those with intervals of more than three years (between first and last endoscopic examinations), the numbers were: a, 17 (68.0%); b, six (24.0%), and c, 2 (8.0%).

When 39 lesions in the a and b subgroups were observed from the standpoint of their first endoscopic findings, 13 showed elevated lesions and 26 depressed lesions, but dysplastic changes (mostly cellular atypia) were visible in the biopsied specimens of the former (10/13) far more frequently than in those of the latter (2/26) (Table 11).

When the same lesions were observed with regard to the histological natures of the cancer, most (9/11) of the cancers with intestinal type histology showed dysplastic changes from the previous biopsied specimens, while none (0/22) were shown by the cancers with diffuse type histology. In the remaining six cases, the relationship between the two findings was not

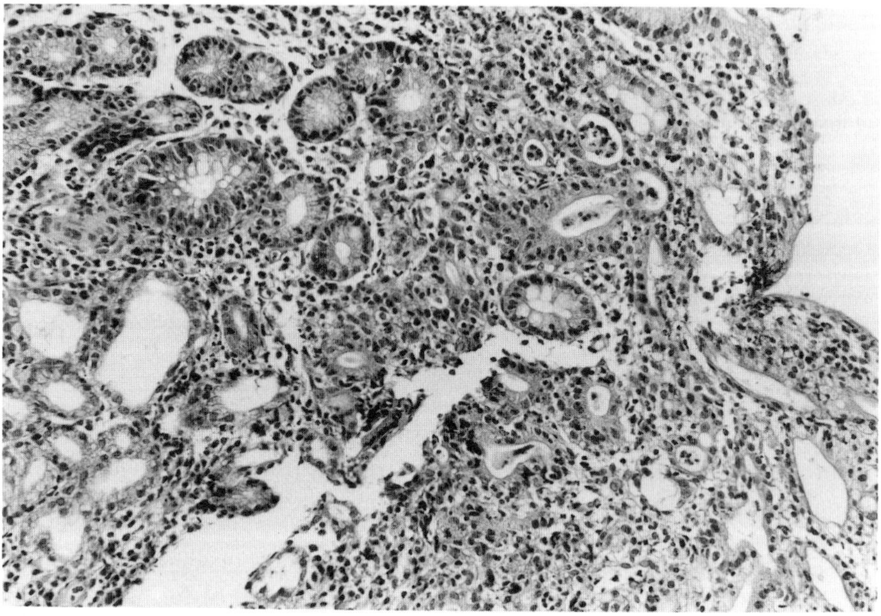

Fig. 7. Minute cancerous change seen in the center of the figure was overlooked at the first biopsy examination, and when the second endoscopic examination was performed 7 years later the cancerous change had progressed significantly

Table 11. Relationship between presence or absence of dysplasia in the *previous* biopsies and of endoscopic follow-up lesions diagnosed as cancer at the *last* biopsy

Biopsy / Endoscop. examination	Dysplasia +	Dysplasia −	Total
Elevated lesion	10	3	13
Depressed lesion	2	24	26
Total	12	27	39

clear owing to the intermediate nature of histology of the cancers (Table 12).

The premalignant nature of the elevated mucosal lesion adjacent to gastrojejunal anastomosis was confirmed by histological examinations of the biopsied specimens taken from 225 lesions with the aid of an endoscope [3].

These results do not necessarily indicate real frequency of precancerous change in the course of development of gastric cancer, as the basic con-

Table 12. Relationship between presence or absence of dysplasia in the *previous* biopsies and of histologic types of the lesions diagnosed as cancer at the *last* biopsy

Biopsy	Dysplasia		Total
Histology	+	–	
Intestinal type	9	2	11
Diffuse type	0	22	22
Others	3	3	6
Total	12	27	39

ditions for the criteria are not fulfilled. In general, however, it can be said that dysplastic changes are more frequently visible in the previous biopsied specimens in the cancers of intestinal type histology than those with diffuse type histology.

Spontaneous development of gastric cancer in elevated lesions through the course of hyperplastic and dysplastic changes has been reported recently in a mutant strain of rodent, Mastomys natalensis [4]. It seems reasonable to suggest, therefore, that some form of precancerous changes – especially in elevated or protruded lesions – is derived from genetical change and is nothing to do with environmental change.

Conclusion

Precursors of the gastric cancer are discussed on the basis of clinical (precancerous conditions) and histological (precancerous lesions) viewpoints and the emphasis is put on the latter.

For the purpose approaching to the subject, surgically resected and endoscopically biopsied specimens were used and "severe dysplasia" was taken as the histological standard.

Even with retrospective follow-up examination of the biopsied gastric lesions, it is still uncertain whether gastric cancers which develop through the precancerous changes belong to minor or major groups. However, in the study described here it seemed necessary, if progress was to be made, to classify gastric cancers into two main types – elevated or depressed, and intestinal or diffuse type histology. This was because the atypical and dysplastic natures of the mucosae are more clearly and more frequently visible in the mucosal lesions with intestinal metaplasia than those without metaplasia.

References

1. Kondo K, Suzuki H, Nagayo T, Yokoyama Y (1982) Pathology of stump carcinoma of the stomach (in Japanese). Gan No Rinsho 28:1615–1623
2. Kondo K, Suzuki H, Nagayo T (1984) The influence of gastro-jejunal anastomosis on gastric carcinogenesis in rats. Gan 75:362–369
3. Kondo K, Kikuchi M, Yokoyama I, Yokoyama Y, Nagayo T (1987) Development of stump carcinoma of the stomach from the viewpoint of biopsied specimens taken from gastric mucosa adjacent to the anastomosis (in Japanese). Gan No Rinsho 33:651–660
4. Kumazawa H, Takagi H, Sudo K, Nakamura W, Hosoda S (1989) Adenocarcinoma and carcinoid developing spontaneously in the stomach of mutant strains of Mastomys natalensis. Virchows Arch [A] 416:141–151
5. Ming SC, Bajtai A, Correa P, Elster K, Jarvi O, Munoz N, Nagayo T, Stemmermann GN (1984) Gastric dysplasia. Significance and pathologic criteria. Cancer 54:1794–1801
6. Morson BC, Sobin LH, Grundmann E, Johansen A, Nagayo T, Serck-Hanssen A (1980) Precancerous conditions and epithelial dysplasia in the stomach. J Clin Pathol 33:711–721
7. Nagayo T (1971) Histological diagnosis of biopsied gastric mucosa with special reference to that of borderline lesions. Gann Monogr Cancer Res 11:243–249
8. Nagayo T (1981) Dysplasia of the gastric mucosa and its relation to the precancerous state. Gan 72:813–823
9. Nagayo T (1983) Precancerous changes of the stomach from the aspect of dysplasia of the gastric mucosa – histological study. In: Sherlock P, Morson BC, Barbara L, Veronesi U (eds) Precancerous lesions of the gastrointestinal tract. Raven, New York, pp 115–126
10. Nagayo T (1986) Gastric cancer preceded by severe dysplasia. Histol Histopathol 1:171–180
11. Nagayo T (1986) Histogenesis and precursors of human gastric cancer. Research and practice. Springer, Berlin Heidelberg New York
12. Nagayo T, Suzuki R, Sato T, Suchi T (1987) Retrospective histoloigcal studies on biopsied gastric lesions of patients in whom cancer was diagnosed at follow-up examination. Jpn J Cancer Res (Gan) 78:995–1005

8 DNA Distribution in Gastric Cancer and Dysplasia

A. Böcking, S. Biesterfeld, and S. Liu

Introduction

During the past few decades some progress has been achieved in the diagnosis and treatment of gastric cancer and its precursors. The development of gastroscopic biopsy, for example, has helped us to achieve earlier diagnosis of gastric carcinoma. Using the information that has been gathered from clinical TNM staging and histopathological features like growth pattern [22] or cellular differentiation [62, 81], internationally acknowledged strategies for gastric cancer surgery have been developed. However, several important diagnostic problems are not fully solved. Two of them reflect the limitations of the subjective microscopic evaluation of tissue specimens:

1. The lack of morphological criteria which would enable use to decide whether a so-called dysplastic lesion is biologically benign or will proceed to morphologically obvious cancer ("prospective malignancy").
2. The insufficient reproducibility of subjective grading systems for dysplasia or carcinoma of 60%–70% [19, 20, 23, 60, 74, 88, 89].

The histological finding of dysplasia does not describe a separate biological entity. Different grades of dysplasia merely reflect different probabilities that a lesion will develop into manifest cancer. The morphological criteria for different grades of dysplasia are ill-defined and subjective, and the results depend very much on the pathologist's experience. Thus, grading results of dysplasia are insufficiently reproducible. However, identification of the obligatory precancerous lesions among the cases of dysplasias would result in early diagnosis of the malignancies.

Another difficult subject has been grading of tumor malignancy. Since investigations of interobserver agreement have shown a reproducibility rate of 60%–70% in, for example, breast carcinoma [19, 23], non-Hodgkin lymphoma [60], prostatic carcinoma [89], urothelial bladder carcinoma, and osteoclastoma [88], every third subjective grading of a malignant tumor will

Institute of Pathology, Aachen University of Technology, Pauwelsstraße 30, W-5100 Aachen, FRG
Cancer Institute, China Medical University, Shenyang, P.R. China

Ying-Chan Zhang/Keiichi Kawai (Eds.)
Precancerous Conditions and Lesions of the Stomach

be wrong. This means that no therapeutic decision should be based on subjective grading results.

Therefore, we need diagnostically and prognostically more relevant parameters which can be objectively and reproducibly quantified if we are to arrive at more reliable diagnoses [87]. During the past few years, especially, DNA cytometric parameters have proven to be of additional diagnostic and prognostic value in different organs and tumors [8, 9, 14, 21, 36, 84]. However, so far there has been no standardization in terminology referring to interpretation of DNA cytometric data. Thus, results from different studies are difficult to compare, and critical evaluation of the worth of diagnostic DNA cytometry is also difficult.

Cytogenetic Background of Diagnostic DNA Cytometry

Nuclei of normal somatic cells contain two sets of 23 chromosomes during the G0/G1 phase of their cell cycle (= 2c). During the G2 phase four sets of chromosomes are present in each nucleus (= 4c). The resulting DNA histogram reveals two peaks corresponding to the G0/G1 and the G2/M phase. The values in between belong to the S phase of the cell cycle. In some tissues a regular multiplicity of this normal chromosomal set can be observed, according to the integer valued exponents of 2c (4c, 8c, 16c), called euploid polyploidization. This polyploidization has for example been observed in mesothelial, urothelial, and seminal vesicle cells, thyrocytes, hepatocytes, and myocardiocytes [12]. Numerical or structural aberrations of these normal chromosomal constitutions are called chromosomal aneuploidy. Chromosomal aneuploidy, which is different from the rest of the somatic cells of an individuum, has only been observed in neoplasms. Thus chromosomal aneuploidy serves as a marker for neoplastic cells in humans [48]. Chromosomal aneuploidy occurs very early in the multistage process of carcinogenesis and precedes the debut of clinical manifestations by many years. Most evidence indicates that the tumor-specific primary chromosomal abnormalities are a prerequisite for carcinogenesis. Chromosomal analysis thus allows the early diagnosis of neoplasia.

Three types of chromosomal abnormalities may be distinguished during tumor progression:

1. Primary, nonrandom, mostly discrete changes preferentially involving specific chromosomes, often as characteristic structural or numerical aberrations. The specificity of these aberrations may allow the diagnosis of certain tumor types. A trisomy of chromosomes 7 and 17, for example, is specific for papillary renal tumors [59]. The detection of cells with aneuploid chromosomal sets is thus equivalent to the detection of neoplastic cells. The resulting DNA histogram mostly reveals a stemline near or at 2c. Thus the effect of primary chro-

mosomal changes on DNA content is mostly not detectable by cytometry.

2. Secondary nonrandom aberrations may follow early during tumor progression. They represent more or less regular additional changes like loss or gain of certain chromosomes and/or, often, an aneuploid polyploidization. These phenomena are associated with a worsening of the patient's prognosis [38]. The changes result in characteristic, clearly abnormal DNA distribution patterns and the appearance of stemlines significantly different from the normal 2c value. The effect of secondary chromosomal aberrations on nuclear DNA content is mostly detectable by cytometry and may serve as an early marker of neoplastic transformation.
3. Tertiary, more massive, random abnormalities affecting all chromosomes equally occur as epiphenomena in later stages of tumor progression. They are observed in addition to primary and secondary aberrations. The more heterogeneous these aberrations are in different cells, the greater is the malignant potential of the tumor [75]. The resulting DNA distribution patterns are characterized by a loss of stemlines and a wide scatter of values. These phenomena merge into one another.

Yet, not the discipline of tumor cytogenetics itself but that of DNA cytometry has used aneuploidy as a marker for neoplastic cell transformation and its extent for grading the malignant potential of various tumors. Slight chromosomal aneuploidies (resulting from primary and secondary aberrations) may often not be detected cytometrically in individual cells because of a limited resolution of the method. A trisomy of chromosomes 7 and 17, for example, results in an increase of total nuclear DNA of 4%, equivalent to 2.08c. But such a small increase may be identified measuring hundreds of cells, statistically comparing their DNA values with those of tissue and individual specific reference cells. This procedure is known as "stemline interpretation of DNA aneuploidy" [2, 37, 73]. So far, a fixed threshold of 2.2c, not considering different CVs of reference and analysis cells, has mostly been used to classify a DNA stemline as aneuploid [6].

We classify a DNA stemline as aneuploid if a statistical comparison of the G0/G1 population of reference cells and analysis cells reveals a p-value of less than 0.001 using the Kolmogorov-Smirnov test [55]. Using that interpretation mode the quantitative effect of minor numerical aberrations (gain or loss of two chromosomes e.g.) on nuclear DNA content may be cytometrically detected.

Single cells from tissues without polyploidization may be identified as aneuploid if their DNA content amounts to more than 4c plus the error of the method. In practice, a DNA content over 5c has been shown empirically to be diagnostically relevant [11, 78]. Not the percentage of cells with a DNA content over 5c, which can be subjectively influenced, but rather their absolute occurrence is of diagnostic relevance (5c exceeding events) [12]. If a polyploidization up to 4c occurs in the given tissue and cells up to 8c in G2/M phase will occur accordingly, the 9c exceedings events may be of diagnostic relevance [24]. We call this procedure "single cell interpretation of DNA aneuploidy". It is sensitive for the detection of single neoplastic cells with an increased aneuploid DNA content, which are present in many malignant tumors.

Both modes of diagnostic DNA data interpretation for the cytometric detection of aneuploidy are correct and should be used in combination, as their sensitivity is complementary.

As the primary, secondary and tertiary chromosomal aneuploidies are specific for most tumors, it is unlikely that one mode of prognostic histogram interpretation or one prognostic DNA index will be valid for a wide range of tumors. Instead, in analogy to morphology, the mode of prognostic DNA data interpretation may be different for each tumor entity. A subjective DNA histogram interpretation prognostically valid for cancers of the breast may not be valid for renal cancers, or a DNA grade of malignancy valid for renal cancers may not be valid for chronic myelogenous leukemias. The relevant mode of diagnostic DNA data interpretation has to be elaborated on the basis of the knowledge about primary, secondary and tertiary chromosomal abnormalities observed in a specific tumor entity. The validity of the prognostic DNA data interpretation has to be established by follow-up studies.

For prognostic interpretation the simple differentiation into "DNA diploid" and "DNA aneuploid" tumors has to be abandoned as it lacks a cytogenetic basis. Nearly all tumors are cytogenetically aneuploid but this may not be detectable by DNA cytometry. Instead, the statistical detection of a DNA aneuploid cell population serves as a marker for neoplasia (see above). For grading purposes the degree of aneuploidy should be quantified either by identification of tumor-specific stemlines [1, 93] or by parameters reflecting the prognostically relevant distribution patterns such as mean ploidy [86], 5c exceeding rate [15], DNA grade of malignancy [13], standard deviation of ploidy [49], and entropy [3, 40, 88].

Chromosomal Changes in Gastric Cancer

Few data are available concerning karyotypic changes in gastric cancer [82]. In a cytogenetic analysis of nine gastric and lower esophageal adenocarcinomas Rodriguez et al. [80] detected nonrandom rearrangements involving the region 11p13–15 on chromosome 8. They thus identified for the first time a specific chromosomal lesion in these tumors. It has been suggested that genetic changes affecting the 11p13–15 region, which were also observed in other tumors, may involve loss of a suppressor gene function. These minor, primary chromosomal aberrations do not result in a significant change of total nuclear DNA. Yet secondary and tertiary aberrations, which follow during tumor progression, mostly are of such extent that a cytometrically detectable increase in total nuclear DNA results [72]. For example, Ochi et al. [70] reported clonal chromosomal abnormalitics in all fivc gastric cancers studied. The genomic rearrangements were numerous; 67 different numerical and 83 different structural changes were seen. The most frequent numerical aberrations were gain of chromosome 12 and loss of Y chromosome. Festi-Passantouopoulou et al. [33] reported trisomies 7, 8, and 9 and structural aberrations of chromosomes 1, 4, and 12. The presence of 49 chromosomes, as described in gastric cancers by Festi-Passantounopoulou et al. [33] and Grauberg et al. [41], results in a modal DNA value of about 2.13c. This increase in modal DNA may be detected cytometrically as significantly different from normal diploid cells (2.0c). As similar numerical changes of chromosomes were so far not described in nonneoplastic gastric mucosa but only found in gastric cancer their DNA cytometric equivalent may be taken as an early marker of neoplasia in gastric dysplasias.

Preparation and Staining

In principle, every type of tissue or cell material may be subjected to single cell DNA cytometry, regardless of its prefixation and staining. Fresh, air-dried smears should be fixed in buffered 4% formaldehyde solution before Feulgen staining with parafuchsine [24]. Differently prestained smears may be uncovered in xylene, postfixed in formaldehyde and restained according to Feulgen [34, 42], even after many years. Destaining will automatically be performed during acid hydrolysis with HCl. Cells may also be released for DNA measurements from old formalin-fixed and paraffin-embedded tissue blocks using cell separation techniques [30]. DNA measurements on sections are allowed only under certain premises: an individual mathematical correction of integrated optical density (IOD) values has to be performed, taking the thickness of the sections and the size of each individual nucleus into account [44]. Correct determination of modal stemline ploidies are not possible measuring on sections. A minimum of 250 cells should be measured to obtain representative results [69]. Material for DNA flow cytometry has to be subjected to special cell separation techniques [7] and stained with fluorescent dyes [94].

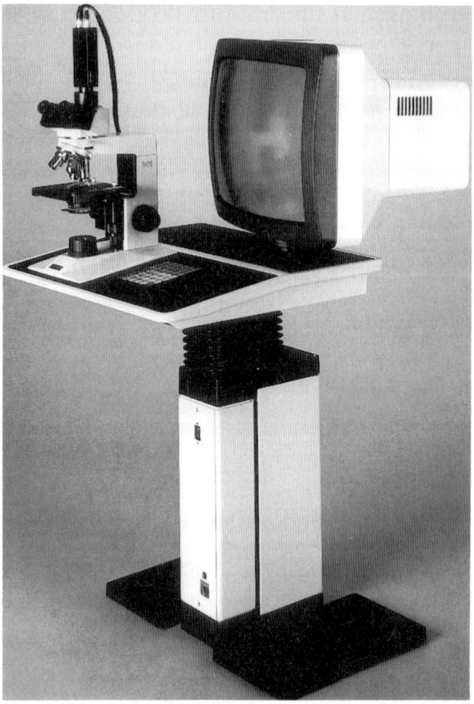

Fig. 1. TV image analysis system combined with a microscope (Cytometer CM1, Hund, Wetzlar, FRG) as an example of equipment for diagnostic DNA single cell cytometry

Equipment for DNA Cytometry

Two different methods are in current use for nuclear DNA quantification: TV-based single cell cytometry and flow cytometry. Each of these methods has advantages and disadvantages which make them suitable for particular diagnostic applications.

TV Image Analysis Systems

TV image analysis systems (Fig. 1) allow single cell DNA measurements on Feulgen-stained cytological routine specimens. Precise DNA measurements for individual cells are obtainable only with single cell cytometry and not with flow cytometry. The cells in question receive exclusive attention; they are morphologically typed and classified as normal, dysplastic or malignant and are measured in a way which prevents their contamination by other cell types. Furthermore, special attention can be paid to the detection of nuclei with defined DNA contents, for example those whose DNA content exceed that in the G2/M phase; this may occur only rarely, but may be of major diagnostic interest ("rare event detection"). A disadvantage, however, is

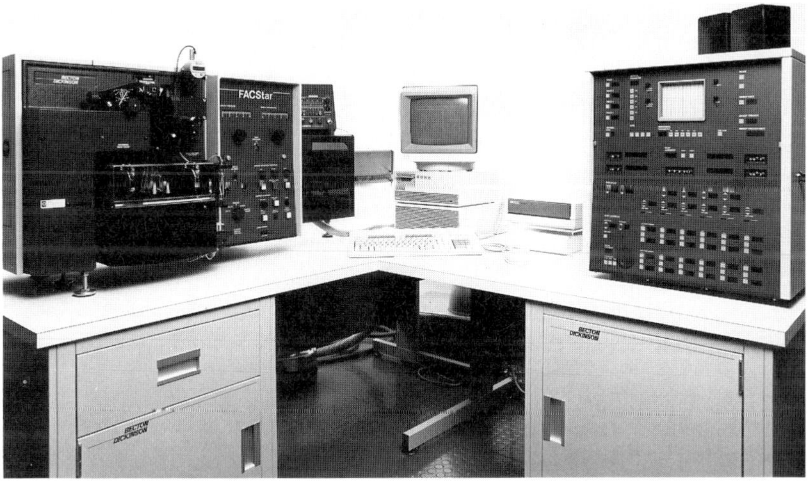

Fig. 2. FACStar (Becton-Dickinson, Mountain View, California, USA) as an example of a flow cytometer will cell sorter

that the number of nuclei measured is limited in comparison with flow cytometry (about 250 per sample). Special attention must be paid to the reference cell system used for DNA cytometry. Only cells with a known DNA content, e.g., lymphocytes, granulocytes, fibroblasts or epithelial cells, which have undergone exactly the same fixation and staining procedures, should be used as individual and tissue-specific reference cells. Because different fixation and preparation procedures have quite different effects on Feulgen hydrolysis, resulting in different staining intensities, the adding of, for example, unfixed blood cells to alcohol-fixed bioptic material or prefixed trout erythrocytes to routine formalin-fixed tumor cells is not allowed [20]. Furthermore, as the stainability of lymphocytes is lower than that of granulocytes and epithelial cells, a preparation- and fixation-specific correction factor, taking differences in laboratory standards into account, has to be introduced [20]. However, details of fixation and preparation procedures, correction factors and quality control of the reference cells used are insufficiently described in most publications. Only reference cells revealing a coefficient of variation of their integrated optical densities below 5% should be used for calibration of the normal 2c value.

Flow Cytometers

Flow cytometers (Fig. 2) allow the rapid DNA quantification of a large number of nuclei in suspension after fluorescence staining. However, the morphologic identification and classification of individual cells is impossible.

Therefore, it might not be possible to differentiate the cells to be measured from lymphocytes, fibroblasts, surrounding normal epithelial cells, and cell clusters. Additionally, only subpopulations representing about 1% or more of the total population can be identified. Thus, rare event detection of a few aneuploid cells in, for example, a fine needle aspiration biopsy is not possible. It might be difficult to decide which channel represents the normal 2c value if no special reference cell system can be used. Several studies on flow cytometry lack information on this important issue.

DNA Cytometric Results in Gastric Mucosa

If aberrations from normal DNA distribution patterns should be interpreted for diagnostic or prognostic purposes, normal gastric mucosa has to be investigated first. Further, changes of DNA distribution in nonneoplastic benign lesions or benign tumors have to be analyzed. Later, the DNA changes of facultative or obligatory precancerous lesions and malignant tumors have to be described.

Normal Gastric Mucosa

In comparison with investigations of other epithelial tissues, among which few or even none are concerned with normal tissue, a surprisingly high number of studies on DNA distribution in normal gastric mucosae have been published [8, 10, 25, 26, 29, 31, 39, 45, 51, 53, 61, 67, 71, 76, 77, 91, 97].

Of the cells, 86%–99% were found in G0/G1 phase near the 2c value; 0.5%–11% were found to be in S phase, corresponding to a usually low proliferative activity. Liu et al. [63] found no cells with a DNA content above 5c and no aneuploid stemline in 32 normal gastric epithelia.

Benign Nonneoplastic Lesions

In cases of *superficial gastritis* only a slight increase in proliferative activity (up to 15%) [29, 97] was described. No "nondiploid" stemline was observed [77, 91, 92].

Nonatrophic chronic gastritis has also been identified as a disease with "diploid" DNA distribution patterns, in some cases combined with an increased percentage of S phase cells. However, it is possible that in some cases cells with DNA content above 4c were recognized [96].

Investigating specimens from the different types of gastritis, Liu et al. [63] identified cells with a DNA content above 5c in 17 out of 30 cases, if these rare events were specifically looked for, with no aneuploid DNA stemline. Similarly in 5 out of 32 cases of "intestinal metaplasia" cells >5c were found but no aneuploid stemline.

So-called *benign ulcer* (a gastric ulcer without any histological sign of dysplasia or other malignancy) has also exhibited a diploid DNA distribution pattern [29, 61, 67, 91]. Cells with DNA contents above 4c corresponding to euploid polyploidization were not observed [61].

Lesions of Uncertain Benignity/Malignancy

Specimens of *chronic atrophic gastritis* generally display proliferative activity approximately 15% greater than that in inflammatory gastric mucosa [29, 96]. Mostly diploid stemlines were found [71, 91, 96]. However, a nondiploid stemline was reported in 11 cases [91, 96], reflecting the possibility of malignant transformation of the epithelial cells. Unfortunately, the resources for sufficient follow-up of all of these cases were not available in three of the patients who underwent control biopsies. Nondiploid populations were repeatedly detectable, and in one case an early cancer was diagnosed after some months. This showed that, at least in one case, proof of a consecutive carcinoma could be demonstrated. The DNA cytometric results of the other ten cases may be interpreted as showing "prospective malignancy"; the histopathological diagnosis of a malignant tumor may be possible within a long follow-up period. Of interest also is the observation that in several cases nondiploid DNA distributions were found in specimens of chronic atrophic gastritis in the areas surrounding histologically proven carcinoma [91]. This finding of DNA aneuploidy underlines the strength of the assumption that malignant alteration may be diagnosed earlier by means of DNA cytometry than by histology alone, as these areas neighboring carcinomas have to be interpreted as histologically not obviously malignant tissues.

In *hyperplastic polyps* diploid distribution pattern was found in combination with an increased proliferation activity of 8%–30%, and the facultative finding of nuclei with DNA content above 4c [31, 77].

Dysplasia represents a major problem in the histopathological diagnosis of gastric lesions. The first reports on DNA cytometric changes in dysplastic tissue of the stomach were published by Macartney and Camplejohn [67]; in 5 out of 16 cases of different grades of dysplasia a nondiploid stemline was detected corresponding to an aneuploid DNA distribution and prospective malignancy. Unfortunately, no follow-up details were available, so the development of a malignant tumor could not be proven.

Recently, our group performed an investigation of 43 cases of gastric dysplasia diagnosed from biopsy specimens in cooperation with the Cancer Institute of the China Medical University, Shenyang, China [64]. For all patients the results of control biopsies relating to a follow-up period of 1–13 years were available. As aneuploid DNA stemlines were not observed in normal gastric mucosa and benign lesions, were chose the statistically significant detection of an aneuploid stemline population ($p < 0.001$, Kolmogorov-Smirnov test) in gastric dysplasias as a marker for prospective malignancy.

Measurements of 200 dysplastic nuclei were performed on cytological specimens prepared from formalin-fixed, paraffin-embedded biopsies by a cell separation technique [30] using a TV image analysis system [4], in combination with an automated microscope (MIAMED, Leica, Wetzlar) [4, 18]. At least 20 lymphocytes from the same specimen served as an internal standard for arriving at the normal 2c level. The DNA cytometric results were compared with the histological diagnoses of the initial biopsy and the control biopsy. Out of 24 cases in which later a carcinoma was diagnosed histologically, 17 were diagnosed by DNA cytometry as prospective malignancy (DNA aneuploid) (Figs. 3, 4). This represents sensitivity to prospective malignancy of 71%, compared with 0% sensitivity by conventional histopathology. In 5 of the 7 false-negative cases the period of time between the biopsy under investigation and the detected carcinoma was short, and a sampling error may have been responsible for the negative diagnosis. In the remaining two cases, in which the carcinoma was diagnosed after 6 or 12 years, there may have been very slight changes in the DNA distribution that were undetectable by DNA cytometry. Of the 19 cases of dysplasia in which cancer did not develop during the follow-up, 18 showed a nonaneuploid DNA stemline, corresponding to a specificity for prospective benignity of 95%.

Gastric Carcinoma

Various studies of DNA distribution in gastric adenocarcinoma revealed diploid stemlines [5, 10, 25–27, 35, 45–47, 52, 61, 67, 68, 76, 85, 90–92, 95–97] or corresponding rates of low ploidy histograms [43, 54, 56–58] in over 80% of cases. Some authors reported frequent occurrence of nuclei with DNA content above the G2/M phase level of 4c in these specimens [25, 31, 97]. On the other hand, nondiploid stemlines as an expression of aneuploidy have been detected in 20%–100% of cases [5, 10, 25–28, 35, 43, 45–47, 52, 54, 56–58, 61, 67, 68, 72, 76, 85, 90–92, 95–97] their values ranging between 2.1c and 4.8c. In one single case a hypodiploid stemline corresponding to a possible chromosomal loss was reported [52]. However, in this case lymphocytes from a lymph node preparation on a different slide were regarded as a reference system, which is now considered unacceptable. Surprisingly, gastric carcinomas of the intestinal type more often revealed severe aberrations from the normal DNA distribution than those of the diffuse type. Nondiploid stemlines were observed in 85%, 77%, 71%, 62%, and 31% of the cases of intestinal carcinoma. We detected DNA aneuploid

Medizinische Fakultät der RWTH Aachen
Institut für Pathologie
Univ.-Prof. Dr. med. Alfred Böcking
Pauwelsstraße 30
D 5100 Aachen

Aachen, 11/18/91

D N A - C Y T O M E T R Y

Filename: C:\USR\CYTO\LUI\LD38.FEX
Patient's name:

Morphological diagnosis: DII
Remarks:

DNA-INTERPRETATION: non aneuploid.

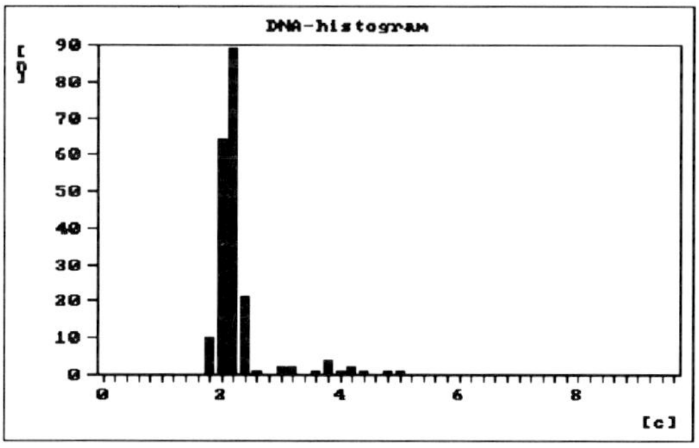

Cytometric parameters:

Number of cells [n]:	200	2c-Deviation Index [c^2]:	0.32
Stemline ploidy [c]:	2.16	Diploid Deviation Quotient:	2.31
DNA index:	1.10	Entropy of DNA:	3.01
5c Exceeding Events [n]:	0	Mean ploidy [c]:	2.26
Aneuploidy Events d [n]:	0	Mean area [μm^2]:	31.34

The statement on DNA-aneuploidy is based on the DNA-stemline interpretation according to Böcking, 1991 ($p<0.001$, Kolmogoroff-Smirnow test). 200 tumor cells were measured at random.

For research use only! This report is not intended for use as a diagnostic procedure without confirmation of the diagnosis by an other medically established diagnostic product or procedure.

Böcking
....
physician's signature

Fig. 3. "Diagnostic letter" of a TV image cytometric measurement of a specimen with moderate dysplasia (DII) from a gastric mucosa with a DNA diagnosis of "nonaneuploid" (stemline ploidy 2.16c). Follow-up: histological diagnosis of mild dysplasia in a control biopsy after 21 months

stemlines in 85% of 34 intestinal carcinomas [65]. Nondiploid stemlines were observed in only 14%, 65%, 20%, 53%, and 17% of the cases of diffuse carcinoma in the same studies [5, 25, 27, 45, 68]. We found aneuploid DNA stemlines in 71% of 63 cases of diffuse types of gastric cancer [63]. A relationship between the histomorphological grading and DNA distribution patterns was found: 36% nondiploidy in G1/G2 tumors and 75% in G3 tumors [26].

Medizinische Fakultät der RWTH Aachen Aachen, 11/18/91
Institut für Pathologie
Univ.-Prof. Dr. med. Alfred Böcking
Pauwelsstraße 30
D 5100 Aachen

D N A - C Y T O M E T R Y

Filename: C:\USR\CYTO\LIU\LD23.FEX
Patient's name:

Morphological diagnosis: DII
Remarks:

DNA-INTERPRETATION: aneuploid.

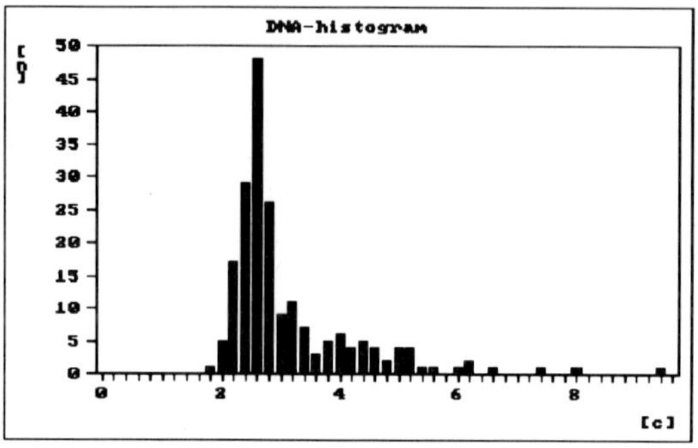

Cytometric parameters:

Number of cells [n]:	200	2c-Deviation Index [c²]:	2.86
Stemline ploidy [c]:	2.60	Diploid Deviation Quotient:	3.17
DNA index:	1.28	Entropy of DNA:	4.59
5c Exceeding Events [n]:	17	Mean ploidy [c]:	3.17
Aneuploidy Events d [n]:	4	Mean area [μm²]:	22.50

The statement on DNA-aneuploidy is based on the DNA-stemline interpretation according to Böcking, 1991 (p<0.001, Kolmogoroff-Smirnow test). 200 tumor cells were measured at random.

For research use only! This report is not intended for use as a diagnostic procedure without confirmation of the diagnosis by an other medically established diagnostic product or procedure.

Böcking
....
physician's signature

Fig. 4. "Diagnostic letter" of a TV image cytometric measurement of a specimen with moderate dysplasia (DII) from a gastric mucosa with a DNA diagnosis of "aneuploid" (stemline ploidy 2.60c). Follow-up: histologically proven gastric adenocarcinoma after 26 months

The few reports in which comparisons with TNM staging have been made indicate that a higher degree of aberration from normal DNA distribution can be found in advanced cancer [35, 57, 83, 85].

A 1-year survival analysis performed on 36 surgically treated patients with adenocarcinomas revealed an overall survival rate of 56% [26]. In general, the survival rate for patients with diploid and nondiploid stemlines amounted to 75% and 38% respectively. In 17 cases of early cancer (survival rate 77%) all 10 patients with a diploid stemline survived (100%), in comparison with only 3 of 7 patients with a nondiploid stemline (43%). In 19 cases of advanced gastric cancer (survival rate 42%) 5 patients of 10 with a diploid stemline (50%) survived 1 year, compared with 3 of 9 patients with a nondiploid stemline (33%).

Survival analysis of 79 cases of gastric adenocarcinoma in a follow-up period of up to 42 months revealed a significantly poorer prognosis for patients with both nondiploid stemlines and increased proliferative activity [90].

Five-year survival rates were determined in a study of 65 surgically treated patients [28]. The survival rate for the whole group was 85%. Independent of any DNA change, all 16 patients with intramucosal lesions were alive (100%). However, in the group of submucosal carcinomas, with an overall survival rate of 80%, 35 of 38 patients (92%) in whom less than 10% of cells had a DNA content above 6c (low ploidy) were alive, compared with 4 of 11 patients (36%) in whom more than 10% of cells had a DNA content above 6c (high ploidy).

Both of these studies were too small to prove the validity of DNA aneuploidy for the prognosis of gastric adenocarcinoma; they did, however, demonstrate that the DNA distribution had a significant influence on the postsurgical prognosis of gastric carcinoma patients. They both gave additional information regarding TNM staging or the infiltration depth of the tumor. These preliminary results are in accordance with those obtained for other malignancies, for example breast carcinoma [19, 32], non-Hodgkin lymphoma [16, 17], renal adenocarcinoma [66, 79], and urothelial bladder carcinoma [50].

Summary

The results of DNA cytometry on various gastric mucosal lesions have been reported in more than 40 publications. We describe the cytogenetic background of diagnostic DNA cytometry and the equipment for its routine application. Normal gastric mucosa is characterized on DNA cytometry by a low proliferative fraction and the absence of cells with a DNA content over 5c. Benign gastritis and intestinal metaplasia reveal diploid DNA stemlines, increased proliferative activity, and few nuclei up to 9c. In gastric dysplasia, aneuploid DNA stemlines are encountered more frequently in those cases in which cancer develops later. An aneuploid DNA stemline in gastric dysplasia may thus serve as an indicator for prospective malignancy (sensitivity 71%, specificity 95%). Gastric cancers exhibit aneuploid DNA stemlines in about 75% of cases, depending on histopathological type, grade of malignancy, and stage. Their DNA distribution may serve as a prognostic index, regardless of clinical staging and histological typing.

References

1. Atkin NB (1976) Prognostic significance of ploidy in human tumors. I. Carcinoma of the uterus. J Natl Cancer Inst 56:909–910
2. Atkin NB, Richards BM (1956) Deoxyribonucleic acid in human tumours as measured by microspectrophotometry of Feulgen stain: a comparison of tumours arising in different sites. Br J Cancer 10:769–786
3. Auer GU, Eriksson E, Azavedo E, Casperson T, Wallgren A (1984) Prognostic significance of nuclear DNA content in mammary adenocarcinomas. Cancer Res 44:394–396
4. Auffermann W, Repges R, Böcking A (1984) Rapid diagnostic DNA cytometry with an automatic microscope and a TV image analysis system. Anal Quant Cytol Histol 6:178–188
5. Ballantyne KC, James PD, Robins RA, Baldwin RW, Hardcastle JD (1987) Flow cytometric analysis of the DNA content of gastric cancer. Br J Cancer 56:52–54
6. Baretton G, Carstensen O, Schardey M, Löhrs U (1991) DNA ploidy and survival in gastric carcinomas: a flow cytometric study. Virchows Arch A 418:301–309
7. Barlogie B (1985) Flow cytometry as a diagnostic and prognostic tool in cancer medicine. In: Büchner et al. (eds) Tumor aneuploidy. Springer, Berlin Heidelberg New York, pp 107–134
8. Barlogie B, Drewinko B, Schumann J, Göhde W, Dosik G, Latreille J, Johnston DA, Freireich EJ (1980) Cellular DNA content as a marker of neoplasia in man. Am J Med 69:195–203
9. Barlogie B, Raber MW, Schumann J, Johnston JS, Drewinko B, Swartzendruber DE, Göhde W, Andreeff M, Freireich EJ (1983) Flow cytometry in clinical cancer research. Cancer Res 43:3982–3997
10. Bennets R, Stroehlein J, Barlogie B (1979) Ploidy determination by DNA flow cytometry of malignant and benign gastric tissue obtained by endoscopic biopsy. Gastroenterology 76:1099
11. Böcking A (1982) Algorithmus für ein universelles DNS-Malignitäts-Grading. Verh Dtsch Ges Pathol 66:540
12. Böcking A (1990) DNA-Zytometrie und Automation in der klinischen Diagnostik. Beitr Onkol 38:298–347
13. Böcking A, Auffermann W (1986) Algorithm for a DNA-cytophotometric diagnosis and grading of malignancy. Anal Quant Cytol Histol 8:383
14. Böcking A, Chatelain R (1989) Diagnostic and prognostic value of DNA cytometry in gynecologic cytology. Anal Quant Cytol Histol 11:177–186
15. Böcking A, Adler CP, Common HD, Hilgarth M, Granzen B, Auffermann W (1984) Algorithm for a DNA-cytophotometric diagnosis and grading of malignancy. Anal Quant Cytol Histol 6:1–7
16. Böcking A, Chatelain R, Auffermann W, Krüger GRF, Asmus B, Wohltmann D, Schuster C (1986) DNA grading of malignant lymphomas. I. Prognostic significance, reproducibility and comparison with other classifications. Anticancer Res 6:1205–1216
17. Böcking A, Chatelain R, Auffermann W, Löhr GW, Reif M, Rossner R, Becker H (1986) DNA grading of malignant lymphomas. II. Correlation with clinical parameters. Anticancer Res 6:1217–1224
18. Böcking A, Sanchez L, Stock B, Müller W (1987) Automated DNA cytometry. Lab Pract 36:73–74
19. Böcking A, Chatelain R, Biesterfeld S, Noll E, Biesterfeld D, Wohltmann D, Goecke C (1989) DNA grading of breast cancer. Prognostic validity, reproducibility and comparison with other classifications. Anal Quant Cytol Histol 11:71–80
20. Böhm N (1968) Einfluß der Fixierung und der Säurekonzentration auf die Feulgen-Hydrolyse bei 28 Grad. Histochemie 15:194–203
21. Böhm N, Sandritter W (1975) DNA in human tumors: cytophotometric study. Curr Top Pathol 60:151–219

22. Borrmann R (1926) Geschwülste des Magens und des Duodenums. In: Henke F, Lubarsch O (eds) Handbuch der speziellen pathologischen Anatomie und Histologie, vol 4. Springer, Berlin Heidelberg New York, p 812
23. Champion HR, Wallace IWJ (1971) Breast cancer grading. Cancer 25:441–448
24. Chatelain R, Hoffmeister B, Härle F, Böcking A, Mittermayer C (1989) DNA grading of oral squamous epithelial carcinomas. A preliminary report. Int J Maxillofac Surg 18:43–46
25. Czerniak B, Herz F, Koss LG (1987) DNA distribution patterns in early gastric carcinomas. Cancer 59:113–117
26. Danova M, Riccardi A, Mazzini G, Wilson G, Dionigi P, Brugnatelli S, Fiocca R, Ucci G, Jemos V, Ascari E (1988) Flow cytometric analysis of paraffin-embedded material in human gastric cancer. Anal Quant Cytol Histol 10:200–206
27. David L, Brandao O, Azavedo RM, Goncalves F, Soares P, Carneiro F, Lopes C, Sobrinho-Simoes M (1989) DNA ploidy pattern of gastric carcinomas. Pathol Res Pract 185:45
28. De Aretxabala N, Yonemura Y, Sugiyama K, Kamata T, Konishi K, Miwa K, Miyazaki (1988) DNA ploidy in early gastric cancer and its relationship to prognosis. Br J Cancer 58:81–84
29. Deinlein E, Schmidt H, Riemann JF, Gräßel-Pietrusky R, Hornstein OP (1983) DNA flow cytometric measurements in inflammatory and malignant human gastric cancer lesions. Virchows Arch A 402:185–193
30. Delgado R, Mikuz G, Hofstädter F (1984) DNA-Feulgen-cytophotometric analysis of single cells isolated from paraffin embedded tissue. Pathol Res Pract 179:92–94
31. Enchev VG, Tsanev KG (1985) Comparative cytomorphometric and cytospectrophometric investigations of gastric lesions. Arch Geschwulstforsch 55:37–46
32. Fallenius A, Franzen S, Auer G (1988) Predictive value of nuclear DNA content in breast cancer in relation to clinical and morphological factors. Cancer 62:521–530
33. Festi-Passantouopoulou AD, Panani AD, Vladios JD, Raptis SA (1987) Common cytogenetic findings in gastric cancer. Cancer Genet Cytogenet 24:63–73
34. Feulgen R, Rossenbeck H (1924) Mikroskopisch chemischer Nachweis einer Nukleinsäure vom Typus der Thymonukleinsäure und die darauf beruhende elektive Färbung von Zellkernen in mikroskopischen Präparaten. Physiol Chem 135:203–247
35. Filipe MI, Sandey A, Costa Rosa J, Imrie P, Ormerod M (1989) DNA content of gastric carcinoma and histological prognostic indices. Pathol Res Pract 185:58
36. Friedlander ML, Hedley DW, Taylor IW (1984) Clinical and biological significance of aneuploidy in human tumours. J Clin Pathol 37:961–974
37. Fu JS, Reagan JW, Richart RM (1981) Definition of precursors. Gynecol Oncol 12:220–231
38. Füzesi L, Zimmermann H, Schaaf UJ, Elbern F, Mittermayer C (1991) Chronologie der zytogenetischen Progression bei Nierenzellkarzinomen. Verh Dtsch Ges Path 75:474
39. Gibel W, Weiß H, Schramm T, Gütz HJ, Wolff G (1972) Untersuchungen über die Möglichkeiten einer Magenkrebsfrüh- und differentialdiagnostik mittels Impulszytophotometrie. Arch Geschwulstforsch 40:263–267
40. Göppinger A, Freudenberg N, Ross A, Hillemanns HG, Hilgarth M (1986) The prognostic significance of the DNA distribution in squamous cell carcinomas of the uterine cervix. Anal Quant Cytol Histol 8:148–151
41. Grauberg I, Gupta S, Zech L (1973) Chromosome analysis of a metastatic gastric carcinoma including quininacrine fluorescence. Hereditas 75:189–194
42. Graumann W (1953) Zur Standardisierung des Schiffschen Reagens. Z Wiss Mikrosk 61:225–226
43. Haraguchi M, Okamura T, Korenaga D, Tsjitani S, Marin P, Sugimachi K (1987) Heterogeneity of DNA ploidy in patients with undifferentiated carcinomas of the stomach. Cancer 59:922–924
44. Haroske G, Dimmer V, Herrmann WR, Kunze KD (1984) Metastasizing APUD cell tumors of the human gastrointestinal tract. Light microscopic and karyometric studies. Pathol Res Pract 178:363–368

45. Hattori T, Hosokawa T, Fukuda M, Sugihara H, Hamada S, Takamatsu T, Nakanishi K, Tsuchiashi Y, Kitamura T, Fujita S (1984) Analysis of DNA ploidy patterns of the gastric carcinomas of Japanese. Cancer 54:1591–1597
46. Hattori T, Hosokawa Y, Sugihara H, Fukuda M, Hamada S, Fujita S (1985) DNA content of diffusely infiltrative carcinomas in the stomach. Pathol Res Pract 180: 615–618
47. Hattori T, Sugihara H, Fukuda M, Hamada S, Fujita S (1986) DNA ploidy patterns of minute carcinomas in the stomach. Jpn J Cancer Res 77:276–281
48. Heim S, Mitelman F (1987) Cancer cytogenetics. Liss, New York
49. Hiddemann W, Schumann J, Andreef M, Barlogie B, Herman CH, Leif RC, Mayall BH, Murphy RF, Sandberg A (1984) Convention on nomenclature for DNA cytometry. Committee on nomenclature, Society for Analytical Cytology. Cancer Genet Cytogenet 13:181–183
50. Hofstädter F, Jakse G, Lederer B, Mikuz G, Delgado R (1984) Biological behaviour and DNA cytophotometry of urothelial bladder carcinoma. Br J Urol 56:289–295
51. Inokuchi K, Koama Y, Sasaki O, Kamegawa T, Okamura T (1983) Differentiation of growth patterns from early gastric carcinoma determined by cytophotometric DNA analysis. Cancer 51:1138–1141
52. Inui W, Oota K (1965) DNA content of human tumor cell nucleus: study on gastric carcinoma, with special reference to its histological features. Jpn J Cancer Res 56:567–574
53. Kamachi M, Morotomi W, Hashimoto T, Fujimoto T, Fujiyama T, Kagawa K, Degushi T, Shimada W, Kodama M, Ashihara T (1984) Cell kinetics and nuclear ploidy pattern in relation to the growth of gastric cancer as analyzed by DNA-RNA cytofluometry. Gan To Kagaku Ryoho 11:2342–2347
54. Kamegawa T, Okamura T, Sugimachi K, Inoruchi K (1986) Preoperative detection of a highly malignant type of early gastric carcinoma by cytophotometric DNA analysis. Jpn J Surg 16:169–1974
55. Kolmogoroff A (1933) Grundbegriffe der Wahrscheinlichkeitsrechnung. Springer, Berlin
56. Korenaga D, Okamura T, Sugimachi K, Inokuchi K (1985) Prognostic study of intramucosal carcinoma of the stomach with DNA aneuploidy. Jpn J Surg 15:443–448
57. Korenaga D, Haraguchi M, Okamura T, Sugimachi K, Kaibara W, Koga S, Inokuchi K (1986) Consistency of DNA ploidy between primary and recurrent gastric carcinomas. Cancer Res 46:1544–1546
58. Korenaga D, Mori M, Okamura T, Sugimachi K, Enoji M (1986) DNA ploidy in clinical malignant gastric lesions less than 5 mm in diameter. Cancer 58:2542–2545
59. Kovacs G, Füzesi L, Emanuel A, Kung HF (1991) Cytogenetics of papillary renal cell tumors. Genes Chromosomes Cancer 3:249
60. Krüger GRF (1983) New Working Formulation für Non-Hodgkin-Lymphome. Eine klinisch-pathologische Korrelation. In: Diehl V, Sack H (eds) Diagnostik und Therapie der Non-Hodgkin-Lymphome. Zuckschwert, Munich (Aktuelle Onkologie, vol 12)
61. Kuwayama H (1979) Feulgen-DNA cytofluorometry and disaccharidase activity in intestinalized gastric mucosa. Gastroenterol Endosc 21:1025–1038
62. Lauren P (1965) The two histological main types of gastric carcinoma: diffuse and so-called intestinal type carcinoma. Acta Pathol Microbiol Scand 64:31–59
63. Liu SQ, Zhang YC, Kropff M, Raupach H, Böcking A (1992) DNA distribution in benign, dysplastic and malignant lesions of the gastric mucosa. Anal Quant Cytol Histol (submitted)
64. Liu SQ, Zhang YC, Kropff M, Böcking A (1991) DNA-Aneuploidy as a marker for prospective malignancy in gastric dysplasias. Pathol Res Pract 187(6):716
65. Liu SQ, Zhang YC, Kropff M, Raupach H, Böcking A (1992) Cytometric evidence for a precancerous lesion of diffuse type gastric cancer: tuboid dysplasia. Am J Clin Pathol (submitted)
66. Ljungberg B, Forsslund G, Stenline R, Zetterberg A (1986) Prognostic significance of the DNA content in renal cell carcinoma. J Urol 135:422–426

67. Macartney JC, Camplejohn RS (1986) DNA flow cytometry of histological materil from dysplastic lesions of human gastric mucosa. J Pathol 150:113–118
68. Macartney JC, Camplejohn RS, Powell G (1986) DNA flow cytometry of histological material from human gastric cancer. J Pathol 148:273–277
69. Marschner S (1992) DNA-Malignitäts-Grading an Mammakarzinom-Feinnadelaspiraten. Dissertation, Technical University of Aachen, FRG
70. Ochi H, Douglass HO Jr, Sandberg AA (1986) Cytogenetic studies in primary gastric cancer. Cancer Genet Cytogenet 22:295–307
71. Odegaard S, Hostmark J, Skagen DW, Schrumpf E, Laerum OD (1987) Flow cytometric DNA studies in normal human gastric mucosa, gastritis and resected stomachs. Scand J Gastroenterol 22:750–756
72. Ojima Y, Inui N, Takeyama S (1962) Studies on the DNA content and the chromosomes in seven cases of human primary gastric carcinoma. Jpn J Cancer Res 53: 123–128
73. Okagaki T, Izuo M (1978) Correction of modal DNA values obtained by microspectrophotometry and tests for their shifts. J Natl Cancer Inst 60:1251–1258
74. Ooms ECM, Kurver PHJ, Veldhuizen RW, Alons CL, Boon ME (1983) Morphometric grading of bladder tumors in comparison with histological grading by pathologists. Hum Pathol 14:144–150
75. Pauwels RPE, Smeets AWGB, Schapers RFM, Geraedts JPM, Debruyne FMJ (1988) Grading in superficial bladder cancer. Cytogenetic classification. Br J Urol 61: 135–139
76. Petrova AS, Subrichina GN, Tschistkova OV, Rottenberg WI, Weiß H, Gütz HJ, Steenbeck L, Wildner GP (1980) Flow cytofluorometry, cytomorphology and histology in gastric carcinoma. Oncology 37:318–324
77. Petrova AS, Subrichina GW, Tschistkova OV, Rottenberg WI, Weiß H, Gütz HJ, Steenbeck L, Wildner GP (1982) Flow cytometry, cytomorphology, histology and autoradiography in human gastric hyperplastic polyps and surrounding mucosa. Oncology 39:308–313
78. Ploem-Zaaijer JJ, Beyer-Boon ME, Leyte Velstra L, Ploem JS (1979) Cytofluorometric and cytophotometric DNA measurements of cervical smears stained using a new bicolor method. In: Pressmann WJ, Wied GL (eds) Automation of cancer cytology and cell image analysis. Tutorials of Cytology, Chicago, pp 225–235
79. Rainwater LM, Hosaka Y, Farrow GM, Lieber MM (1987) Well differentiated clear cell carcinoma: significance of nuclear desoxyribonucleic acid patterns studied by flow cytometry. J Urol 137:15–20
80. Rodriguez E, Rao PH, Ladanyi M, Altorki N, Albino AP, Kelsen DP, Jhanwar SC, Chaganti RSK (1990) 11p13–15 is a specific region of chromosomal rearrangement in gastric and esophageal adenocarcinomas. Cancer Res 50:6410–6416
81. Rotterdam H (1989) Carcinoma of the stomach. In: Rotterdam H, Enterline HT (eds) Pathology of the stomach and duodenum. Springer, Berlin Heidelberg New York, pp 142–204
82. Sandberg AA (1990) The chromosomes in human cancer and leukemia, 2nd ed. Elsevier, New York
83. Sannohe Y, Hiratsuka R (1981) Clinico-pathological significance of the DNA histogram pattern in cancer cell nuclei of the stomach and the esophagus. Gastroenterol Jpn 16:25–32
84. Seckinger D, Sugarbaker E, Frankfurt O (1989) DNA content in human cancer. Arch Pathol Lab Med 113:619–626
85. Sowa M, Yoshino H, Kato Y, Wishimura M, Kamino K, Umeyama K (1988) An analysis of the DNA ploidy patterns of gastric cancer. Cancer 62:1325–1330
86. Sprenger E, Volk L, Michaelis WE (1974) Die Aussagekraft der Zellkern-DNS-Bestimmung bei der Diagnostik des Prostatakarzinoms. Beitr Pathol 153:370–378
87. Stenkvist B, Olding-Stenkvist E (1990) Cytological and DNA characteristics of hyperplasia, inflammation and cancer of the prostate. Eur J Cancer 26:261–267
88. Sun D, Biesterfeld S, Adler CP, Böcking A (1992) Prediction of recurrence in giant cell tumors of the bone by DNA cytometry. Anal Quant Cytol Histol (accepted)

89. Svanholm H, Mygind H (1985) Prostatic carcinoma. Reproducibility of histology grading. Acta Pathol Microbiol Immunol Scand (A) 93:67–71
90. Szentirmay Z, Csuka O, Sugar J (1986) DNA and enzyme histochemistry of dysplasia and gastric cancer. In: Fillipe IM, Jass JR (eds) Gastric carcinoma. Livingstone, Edinburgh, pp 68–86
91. Teodori L, Capurso L, Cordelli E, de Vita R, Koch M, Tarquini M, Pallone F, Mazro F (1984) Cytometrically determined relative DNA content as an indicator of neoplasia in gastric lesions. Cytometry 5:63–70
92. Teodori L, Tirindelli-Danesi D, Cordelli E, Uccelli R, de Vita R, Spano M, Mauro F, Schillaci A, Moraldi A, Capuso L, Stipa S (1984) Potential prognostic significance of cytometrically determined DNA abnormality in GI tract human tumors. Ann New York Acad Sci 291–301
93. Tribukait B (1989) Rapid flow cytometry of prostatic fine needle aspiration biopsies. In: Karr DS, Coffey W, Gardner (eds) Prognostic cytometry and cytopathology of prostate cancer. Elsevier, New York, pp 263–242
94. Vindelöv LL, Christensen J (1989) Some methods and applications of flow cytometric DNA analysis in clinical and experimental oncology. Eur J Haematol [Suppl] 42:69–76
95. Weiß H, Heinz H, Wildner GP (1980) The influence of heparin on DNA distribution patterns of gastric mucosa as obtained by flow cytometry. Preliminary report. Arch Geschwulstforsch 50:119–124
96. Weiß H, Wildner GP, Gütz HJ, Ebeling K, Steinhoff G, Tanneberger S (1981) DNA distribution patterns of preneoplastic cells and their interpretation. Oncology 38: 210–218
97. Wiendl HJ, Schwabe M, Becker G, Kowatsch J (1974) Feulgen-cytophotometric studies of gastric mucosal smears in malignant and benign diseases of the stomach. Acta Cytol 18:222–230

Subject Index